# Autism and Child Psychopathology Series

**Series Editor**
Johnny L. Matson
Louisiana State University, Baton Rouge, USA

**Brief Overview**

The purpose of this series is to advance knowledge in the broad multidisciplinary fields of autism and various forms of psychopathology (e.g., anxiety and depression). Volumes synthesize research on a range of rapidly expanding topics on assessment, treatment, and etiology.

**Description**

The **Autism and Child Psychopathology Series** explores a wide range of research and professional methods, procedures, and theories used to enhance positive development and outcomes for children. Developments in education, medicine, psychology, and applied behavior analysis as well as child development across home, school, hospital, and community settings are the focus of this series. Series volumes are both authored and edited, and they provide critical reviews of evidence-based methods. As such, these books serve as a critical reference source for researchers and professionals who deal with childhood disorders and disabilities, most notably autism, intellectual disabilities, challenging behaviors, anxiety, depression, ADHD, developmental coordination disorder, communication disorders, and other common childhood problems. The series addresses important mental health and development difficulties that children, their caregivers, and the professionals who treat them must face. Each volume in the series provides an analysis of methods and procedures that may assist in effectively treating these childhood problems.

More information about this series at http://www.springer.com/series/8665

Stephanie M. Hadaway • Alan W. Brue

# Practitioner's Guide to Functional Behavioral Assessment

## Process, Purpose, Planning, and Prevention

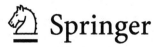 Springer

Stephanie M. Hadaway
Bartow County School System
CARTERSVILLE
Georgia
USA

Alan W. Brue
Bartow County School System
EUHARLEE
Georgia
USA

ISSN 2192-922X                                    ISSN 2192-9238 (electronic)
Autism and Child Psychopathology Series
ISBN 978-3-319-23720-6                            ISBN 978-3-319-23721-3 (eBook)
DOI 10.1007/978-3-319-23721-3

Library of Congress Control Number: 2015950750

Springer Cham Heidelberg New York Dordrecht London

Printed on acid-free paper

Springer International Publishing AG Switzerland is part of Springer Science+Business Media (www.springer.com)

*Stephanie: I would like to dedicate this book to my husband, Lee, who never ceases to amaze me! Thank you for always seeing the best in me.*

*Alan: This book is for my wife, Jett, who is always so very supportive of everything that I do. You are the best!*

# Acknowledgments

We would like to acknowledge and thank the parents, teachers, and administrators with whom we have worked. We have learned a lot from them and have incorporated this knowledge in our daily work with children and adolescents.

# Contents

## Part III   Phase II: Purpose

# About the Authors

**Stephanie M. Hadaway Ed.S., LPC** received her Master of Education in Guidance and Counseling from the University of Tennessee at Chattanooga and her Educational Specialist (Ed.S.) in Educational Leadership from Nova Southeastern University. Ms. Hadaway has a rich background in child and adolescent therapy. As a Licensed Professional Counselor (LPC) in Georgia, she has worked with adults, couples, adolescents, and children with a variety of mental health needs. Specifically, Ms. Hadaway has specialized in serving children and adolescents with severe emotional disturbance in both outpatient and day treatment settings. She has facilitated groups, worked with families, and provided individual therapy. In addition to providing therapeutic counseling services, Ms. Hadaway has spent more than 10 years providing educational and behavioral support within the public school system. She is a certified teacher who has worked in both elementary and middle schools in the inclusive, resource, and self-contained settings. Currently, she is a behavior specialist within the public school system and serves all grade levels.

**Alan W. Brue Ph.D., NCSP** received his Master of Arts, Education Specialist, and Doctor of Philosophy degrees in school psychology from the University of Florida. Dr. Brue is a Nationally Certified School Psychologist (NCSP) who has worked for more than 15 years providing a wide range of school psychological services to metro-Atlanta school districts. He currently works as a school psychologist and has extensive knowledge of and experience with children and adolescents who exhibit behavior problems. In addition to his school-based experience, Dr. Brue currently holds a core faculty teaching position in a school psychology training program, where he develops and teaches graduate classes, such as Functional Behavioral Assessment, Psychopathology of Children and Adolescents, Psychological Assessment, Exceptional Children in the Classroom, and Child and Adolescent Development. With Linda Wilmshurst, he has coauthored *A Parent's Guide to Special Education: Insider Advice on How to Navigate the System and Help Your Child Succeed* (AMACOM 2005), *The Complete Guide to Special Education: Expert Advice on Evaluations, IEPs, and Helping Kids Succeed (Second Edition)* (Jossey-Bass 2010), and *Essentials of Intellectual Disability Assessment and Identification* (Wiley 2016). Dr. Brue's website is AlanBrue.com.

# List of Abbreviations

| | |
|---|---|
| ABA | Applied behavior analysis |
| ABC | Antecedent-behavior-consequence |
| ADHD | Attention-deficit/hyperactivity disorder |
| ASD | Autism spectrum disorder |
| BACB | Behavior Analyst Certification Board |
| BIP | Behavior intervention plan |
| CECP | Center for Effective Collaboration and Practice |
| FAPE | Free Appropriate Public Education |
| FBA | Functional behavioral assessment |
| FERPA | Family Educational Rights and Privacy Act of 1974 (also known as the Buckley Amendment) |
| IDEA 2004 | Individuals with Disabilities Education Improvement Act of 2004 |
| IEP | Individualized Education Program |
| LRE | Least restrictive environment |
| ODD | Oppositional defiant disorder |
| OSEP | Office of Special Education Programs |
| OSERS | Office of Special Education and Rehabilitative Services |
| PBIS | Positive Behavioral Interventions and Supports |
| RTI | Response to Intervention |

# Part I
# Introduction

# Chapter 1
# Introduction to the FBA Process: How to Use This Book

## What You Need to Know

Let us start with what counts. This book is designed for those of you who are *working with* or *learning to work with* individuals exhibiting behaviors that impact their ability to adapt appropriately to their environment. It is designed to be used as a practical application for those directly involved in the classroom, community, or residential setting. You may be a college student, teacher, counselor, school psychologist, residential coordinator, or even a behavior specialist. You may have a lot of experience with individuals exhibiting behavioral difficulties or this may be your very first year working with them. It does not matter. This book is designed to give you a manageable approach to what can be a challenging area. It is based on our collective experiences and has grown from the difficulties we have encountered in our day-to-day professional lives. There are a lot of great ideas and strategies to writing functional behavioral assessments (FBAs) available to the public. We have taken our own needs and reconceptualized how the process should work. Those reflections and experiences are the foundational structure of this book. We want you to take our hard-earned lessons and make your own process much easier.

## Strategy One: Understand the Basics

This book is about sharing a philosophy on how to create an effective FBA. As a point of reference, it is important that we clarify the content in question. One faulty assumption that we often encounter is that FBA and functional analysis are interchangeable terms. FBA is a set of techniques and strategies that are designed to ascertain relational connections between a respondent and environmental conditions. Creating a comprehensive FBA entails both indirect assessment and direct assessment to form a hypothesis regarding the behavior of concern. Functional analysis might be a com-

© Springer International Publishing Switzerland 2016
S. M. Hadaway, A. W. Brue, *Practitioner's Guide to Functional Behavioral Assessment,*
Autism and Child Psychopathology Series, DOI 10.1007/978-3-319-23721-3_1

ponent of this assessment. It is an experimental method designed to test the accuracy of the hypothesis through the manipulation of variables. The appropriateness of its inclusion should be weighed in light of need and accessibility when considering environmental and situational components.

In our experience with behavioral applications, consistency is often linked with effectiveness. It seems to us that those who have achieved a high degree of professional consistency and, subsequently, professional effectiveness have an underlying set of guiding principles. Without a well-understood philosophical and practical base, some are inclined to jump on every new trend or technique often yielding unfruitful progress in their practice. Developing a foundational assumption has helped to steer us towards the applications that are beneficial to those we support.

Our behavioral philosophy rests on several assumptions that guide our practice. First, behavior cannot be viewed in single, isolated episodes. Choosing to let one behavioral incident shape our perceptual understanding of a person is like looking at a photograph taken in 1 s and believing that it defines a person's next 24 h of living. Understanding a person's behavior means looking beyond one or two occurrences of challenging behavior. It requires perspective and just one glance will not suffice. If you are going to obtain a realistic perspective of an individual's behavior, nothing will be as beneficial as viewing the individual multiple times across a landscape that encompasses variability in contextual factors such as those present, setting and events taking place. When an interfering behavior does not occur often yields just as much meaningful data as when it does occur. Therefore, guard against defining the function of an interfering behavior based on an isolated incident.

Second, effective behavioral interventions cannot be overgeneralized. In order for behavior planning to be successful, it must be individualized and cover both deliberate assessment and deliberate prevention. Even good strategies will not work with every person. Therefore, strategies must be driven by data, knowledge, and understanding. If any of those components are lacking, it weakens the strategy.

Finally, FBA is a tool. Just as a hammer is essential in building a house, it is not the only tool needed. It would be very difficult to effectively cut wood with a hammer. And it would be very difficult to hold boards in place without the use of nails. When it comes to understanding and addressing behavioral needs in individuals, there are many evaluative and experiential methods that can be used. When chosen at random or used in isolation, these tools have little effectiveness in the resolution of interfering behaviors. Worse, sometimes the misapplication of a strategy can actually deter progress. Addressing challenging behaviors efficiently requires identifying a person-specific set of behavior planning tools, and working those tools to successfully complement one another. FBA is a useful tool, but it should not be considered a means to an end. Rather, the FBA process is more like the starting point on a behavioral planning map. Once it is completed, it determines the direction that behavior planning will take for an individual. Therefore, it should be approached thoughtfully.

# Strategy Two: Understand the Scope

In order to encompass this type of approach, we decided as practitioners that we needed a fresh way to look at the FBA process. We did this by viewing both the development of an FBA and the creation of a behavioral plan as occurring in four essential phases. These phases are sequential and build on each other. We identified them as *Process, Purpose, Planning,* and *Prevention.*

Process is the beginning phase of FBA. Within Process, the practitioner would make preparations, review records, interview the student and other contributing parties, utilize assessments, collect data, and complete observations. The Process phase could also be considered the *doing* or *working phase*. This phase is about gathering, asking, reviewing, and observing. It is driven by focusing on target behaviors. These behaviors have been defined by the practitioner typically in conjunction with the individual's team. By making the effort to attain good, reliable, and sound information in this phase, the practitioner is prepared to continue to make good, reliable, and sound decisions in the next phase. The groundwork attained in Process is what underlies data analysis and propels decision-making forward. So, this process moves the practitioner into determining the purpose of the exhibited behavior.

Purpose is the second phase. Just as Process needs to be reliable, Purpose needs to be sound. Within Purpose, the practitioner begins data analysis. This involves looking critically at all of the information gathered. It is a detail-oriented task that requires organization and reflection. After analysis, the practitioner uses the results obtained to form a hypothesis about the function of the individual's behavior. If appropriate, functional analysis will begin in order to test the hypothesis. Once the purpose of the exhibited behavior has been defined, the practitioner, often along with a team, can develop a behavior plan.

Planning is the third phase and a step just beyond writing an FBA. Within Planning, the practitioner leads the team in developing interventions based on the hypothesis statement. Interventions include defining replacement behaviors and identifying strategies and curriculum to use. During Planning, reinforcers and consequences are determined based on the individual's personal preferences. Also, an action plan that entails how additional data will be collected on the progress of interventions is enacted. When behavior planning is set into motion, this leads to prevention.

Prevention is the final phase of our multiphasic approach to behavior planning. Within Prevention, the practitioner remains a strong voice but is also a collaborator with the team for the prevention of behaviors. The climate, culture, and community all can equally serve to minimize or increase the demonstration of disruptive behavior. Even with the best Process, Purpose, and Planning in place, a lack of commitment to Prevention as a whole will give rise to behavioral challenges. Without an effort towards prevention, negative and difficult behavior might reemerge despite all other attempts at behavior management.

Ultimately, Process, Purpose, Planning, and Prevention are phases that help us to think about more long-term solutions. For us, this model changes how we teach other professionals about behavior and behavior planning. Our goal is to simplify the process of planning and development. It is our hope that you can turn to any part of this book and understand where you are in the development of an FBA and behavior planning.

## Strategy Three: What to Do

Use this book to its fullest! Dive into these concepts and allow them to anchor your thinking about how to approach behavioral planning. Use the four phases as divisions for clarification. Instead of thinking about them as four distinct points, consider them as four stairs that lead to an informational result. Behavior planning is a comprehensive effort; make this book your jumping-off point.

To aid you in this process, we have used two methods to help make this information applicable to you. First, each chapter has been designed in a consistent format. If you look back through this chapter, the format will become clearer. We have built the structure in a hierarchical manner that takes you from the basics of the presented topic, widens the scope of understanding, tells the practitioner step by step what to do, and then applies the information presented. Subsequently, each chapter ends with a "takeaway" from us, the authors—Stephanie, a behavior specialist, and Alan, a school psychologist. These "takeaway" moments are our individual viewpoints—based on our training and school-based experiences—regarding the content of that chapter. Second, we have added a case snapshot of Willow Wilding to guide you through a generalized application and perhaps inject a measure of levity in the book. This ends with both an FBA and behavior intervention plan in Chap. 12.

Additionally, we encourage you to use the worksheets provided throughout the book. We will be the first to say there are plenty of good ways to approach all of the information that we have provided. In fact, your organization or school district might mandate the use of certain forms. We understand this because we have similar mandates on paperwork. But, if you can, use these forms as you go through the book, if only for practice. They have been especially designed to complement the four-phase model we have developed.

Finally, we have spent a portion of many chapters in this book addressing what we will term, "professional conduct." When called upon to execute the steps in behavior planning, the practitioner will enter into both environmental and relational situations. Technically, your approach may be thorough and exact. You may understand how to successfully apply techniques and strategies to create an exceptional plan. Yet, our experience has taught us that the willingness of organizations and individuals to remain open to this process can be equally enhanced and limited by their interactions with the practitioner. Therefore, we have provided guidelines on how to maintain professional conduct throughout the FBA process.

## Strategy Four: Application

The application of this chapter is twofold. First, we encourage you to read on. As much as we have simplified this information, some of it might still seem challenging. In those moments, take a break and come back to the material fresh. Second, reflect on your own cases as you work through this book. For instance, when we take you step by step through the development of a target behavior, try this yourself. Before you bring this information into practice, it is good to try it privately. You might even want to work through the material with a partner or a group. However you approach the creation of FBA, it is our hope that this book will be an excellent resource for you.

## A Before-You-Proceed Checklist

1. Understand that behavior cannot be viewed accurately in single episodes.
2. Understand that behavior planning must be individualized.
3. Familiarize yourself with the four phases.
4. Understand that FBA is the starting point of behavioral planning.

**Author Takeaways**
*From both Stephanie, the behavior specialist, and Alan, the school psychologist:*

Interfering or inappropriate behaviors are sometimes difficult to understand. They can bring unrest and chaos into any setting. There are many strategies and curricula that are available; however, these have little effectiveness if the purpose of an individual's challenging behavior is unknown. Addressing the right issue with appropriate reinforcements is essential in working towards the resolution of misbehavior. FBA is the tool that aids the practitioner in gaining this information. By the end of this book, we hope you will feel confident in using that tool as needed. Happy reading.

# Chapter 2
# The Basics of Functional Behavioral Assessment

## What You Need to Know

We introduced you to the four-phase concept in Chap. 1. The first phase, *Process*, is the working phase of writing a functional behavioral assessment (FBA). Before beginning, it is vital that you develop an understanding of the language and underlying principles that govern the development of an FBA.

In this chapter, our goal is not to give you an in-depth history of FBA. However, it seems to us that we would be remiss if we jumped straight into the FBA process without offering you an understanding of the theoretical fields from which this tool has emerged. We also felt that those of you working in the field of education should know the regulations that govern the use of FBA in public schools. This chapter might seem a bit heavy, perhaps even wordy. *Do not worry!* This is a practitioner's guide. After you wade through the concepts contained in this chapter, the book will take you step by step through the process of completing an FBA. But, first things first—let us begin.

## Strategy One: Understand the Basics

Over the years, we have read and studied different viewpoints on the ramifications involved in defining FBA. The Center for Effective Collaboration and Practice (CECP) considers FBA to be "a problem-solving process for addressing student problem behavior." They go on to include that this process uses strategies and techniques that lead to understanding the purpose of an individual's behavior. (This is from the helpful CECP website at http://cecp.air.org/fba/. They are funded by the Office of Special Education Programs and several other government agencies.) Our cue is taken from this problem-solving process. As practitioners, we have come to define FBA as a multilayered method of determining the function or intent of a behavior. It is a systemized approach that allows the practitioner to answer the question, "What purpose does this behavior serve?" Within the context of supporting an

© Springer International Publishing Switzerland 2016                                   9
S. M. Hadaway, A. W. Brue, *Practitioner's Guide to Functional Behavioral Assessment,*
Autism and Child Psychopathology Series, DOI 10.1007/978-3-319-23721-3_2

individual with behavioral challenges, the question typically focuses on the aberrant or interfering behavior.

## *Functional Behavioral Assessment and Behaviorism*

Let us rewind the clock now. The FBA approach has a history with deep roots in the fields of learning and behavior. Behaviorism or behavioral psychology is the cornerstone to this vast field of theory, experiment, and application. Behaviorism asserts that behavior is learned. So, what is learned can essentially be unlearned and replaced with alternative behavior. Pioneering research in this field includes works by John B. Watson (1913), Ivan Pavlov (1927), Edward L. Thorndike (1911), and B. F. Skinner (1953).

You might remember from a child development class or a general psychology course the controversial "Little Albert" experiment by John B. Watson. In this study, Watson demonstrated the impact of conditioning on an 11-month-old boy. In brief, the child was presented with a white rat and then an iron rod was loudly clanged causing the child to cry. This process was repeated until the child began to cry when the white rat was presented without an accompanying noise. Subsequently, the boy cried when a white rabbit, a dog, and even fur were presented to him.

Now, what was Watson attempting to do? He was attempting to demonstrate that through the introduction of a stimulus, he could create a specific response. Although controversial, Watson seemed to have successfully "conditioned" the boy to express a fear response. Whenever the 11-month-old was presented with a furry animal or object, he cried. In this regard, Watson appeared to have successfully paired a stimulus (furry animal or object) with a response (crying).

In Watson's day, the popular psychological perspective focused on internal urges. Through his experimental work, Watson was attempting to show that human behavior was not caused by internal drives. He was attempting to establish that environment impacted the formulation of behaviors. This environmental impact could be manipulated to then create a change in the individual. In the journal *Psychological Review,* Watson (1913) wrote:

> Psychology as the behaviorist views it is a purely objective experimental branch of natural science. Its theoretical goal is the prediction and control of behavior. Introspection forms no essential part of its methods, nor is the scientific value of its data dependent upon the readiness with which they lend themselves to interpretation in terms of consciousness. The behaviorist, in his efforts to get a unitary scheme of animal response, recognizes no dividing line between man and brute. (p. 162)

Watson, known as the father of behaviorism, was not the only pioneer in the field. In the area of conditioning, Ivan Pavlov and B. F. Skinner are two key figures. You might remember that conditioning is pairing a stimulus with a response. This should sound somewhat familiar based on the preceding paragraphs. For a brief review and a quick reminder, we will cover the two most basic types of conditioning: classical and operant.

a. *Classical conditioning:*

Ivan Pavlov is probably best known for his conditioning dogs to salivate at the sound of a bell.

Step 1: A naturally occurring stimulus is paired with an unconditioned response.

| *Food* | *Salivation* |
|---|---|
| *Unconditioned stimulus* | *Unconditioned response* |

Step 2: A neutral stimulus is paired with the naturally occurring stimulus.

    *Bell + Food = Salivation*

This is repeated until the neutral stimulus (bell) begins to prompt the unconditioned response (salivation) without the naturally occurring stimulus (food) present.

| *Bell* | *Salivation* |
|---|---|
| *Conditioned stimulus* | *Conditioned response* |

b. *Operant conditioning:*

B. F. Skinner differentiated between a natural response, such as salivation in the presence of food, and a learned response that takes place through both reinforcement and punishment. The respondent begins to link behavior and consequence through operant conditioning. If the respondent finds the consequence desirable or positive, he or she is more likely to repeat the behavior; however, if the respondent finds the consequence too negative or undesirable, he or she is less likely to repeat the behavior. Skinner identified these consequences as reinforcements and punishments. According to Skinner (1953), "The strengthening of behavior which results from reinforcement is appropriately called 'conditioning'. In operant conditioning we 'strengthen' an operant in the sense of making a response more probable or, in actual fact, more frequent" (p. 42).

During the 1950s and the 1960s, many researchers began to move towards developing behavioral change experiments with humans. Numerous studies were completed and an ever-growing body of research was developed. Behavior modification moved to the forefront as experiments demonstrated the impact of consequence on the behavior of human respondents. In the late 1960s, Sidney Bijou began using strategies designed by Skinner. He focused his work in the area of child development. As a result, Bijou was one of several who formalized techniques, such as the antecedent-behavior-consequence (ABC) model. This model allows the observer to gather information to analyze how the antecedent *(what comes before)* and the consequent *(what comes after)* impact the behavior of a respondent. For example, Ms. Mealer passes out the math assignment *(antecedent)*. Aaliyah begins to cry *(behavior)*. Ms. Mealer comforts Aaliyah and helps her answer the first few questions *(consequence)*. Of further impact, Bijou, along with Donald Baer, Todd Risley, James Sherman, and Montrose Wolf, founded the *Journal of Applied Behavior Analysis* in 1968.

Certainly, this brief summary is too limited to detail the many contributions that other researchers and scientists have made. Over the course of decades, the foundational importance of applying behavioral strategies was established. Behavioral modification emerged as a focus to work with the deterrent of unwanted behavior. Although there was great progress in the field, an actual format for conducting an experimental functional analysis was not introduced until 1982, when the influential article by Iwata, Dorsey, Slifer, Bauman, and Richman was published. Dixon et al. (2012) write, "The seminal 1982 paper by Iwata et al. offered an elegant yet powerful format for conducting experimental assessments of the function of maladaptive behaviors, and the three decades that have passed since its publication have seen the basic format used across a variety of other populations, settings, and behaviors." The format outlined in the article is still in use today.

Currently, research and application can be found in the fields of experimental analysis of behavior and applied behavior analysis. Experimental analysis of behavior is the scientific approach to studying the relationship between behavior and environment. As the name implies, it is experimental in nature and takes place in a controlled environment. The Behavior Analyst Certification Board (BACB) defines behavior analysis as "both an applied science that develops methods of changing behavior and a profession that provides services to meet diverse behavioral needs. Briefly, professionals in applied behavior analysis engage in the specific and comprehensive use of principles of learning, including operant and respondent conditioning, in order to address behavioral needs of widely varying individuals in diverse settings" (http://www.bacb.com/index.php?page=2).

In the modern world, perhaps much of this thinking is now commonplace. The influential experiments of Pavlov, Watson, and Skinner are now part of our collective understanding. What was once new and untried is now scientific history. In this day and age, we might have grown accustomed to not just hearing about, but actually using an ABC chart to collect data. Although public schools are not filled with sanitized laboratories stocked with clanging rods and white rats, evidence of behavior change instruments is readily found. Classrooms are filled with reinforcers and consequences, such as sticker charts and changing a student's color based on adherence to classroom rules. It seems then that the proverbial groundwork was substantially laid, and with this, FBA was introduced into the public educational system.

## *Functional Behavioral Assessment and Education*

FBA became an official expectation of the public educational system in 1997 with Public Law 105-17. The Individuals with Disabilities Education Act Amendments of 1997 was the first time an FBA was mandated by the government. In 2004, this law was amended to form the Individuals with Disabilities Education Improvement Act (IDEA) 2004. IDEA 2004 is the current federal law upheld today; it went into effect on July 1, 2005.

So, what does all of this mean? When a student is identified as having a disability, IDEA 2004 gives them certain rights and protections (Wilmshurst and Brue 2010). A child with a disability has a right to a free appropriate public education (FAPE) and to be educated in the least restrictive environment (LRE). Students who exhibit challenging behaviors are more likely to have more restrictive placements in school when compared to peers (Becker et al. 2011; Bradley et al. 2008; Sanford et al. 2011; Smith et al. 2011). LRE is the legal guarantee that when a student's placement is considered, he or she will be educated with their nondisabled peers to the greatest degree that is appropriate. As part of federal law, a child with a disability has an individualized education program (IEP) that is developed annually. If a student with a disability is found to have behaviors that impede his or her learning or the learning of others, the IEP team must consider the development of a behavior intervention plan (BIP). The BIP needs to include positive behavior supports and interventions. Although IDEA 2004 does not mandate the format or requirements of a BIP, effective plans often include interventions, reinforcers, and consequences. One significant benefit to adding a BIP is that once it has been developed by an IEP team, it is a legal document. Furthermore, it mandates a measure of uniformity and consistency in which everyone who works with the student will respond to the identified target behavior.

Let us pause here for just a moment. Do not worry—if this is a lot of information to digest, we are going to cover this territory again. In fact, Chap. 13 is all about writing BIPs. For now, it is important to understand that if a student with a disability has interfering behaviors, the student's IEP team has the responsibility to consider the development of a BIP. Let us emphasize the word *consider*.

In order for a BIP to be effective, the team needs to understand the interventions and strategies necessary for behavior change. Each child is different, and strategies need to be individualized. Even successful strategies do not work with everyone. How does the IEP team know what to address in the BIP? The best way to determine this is to complete an FBA. As noted, we define an FBA as a multilayered method of determining the function or intent of a behavior. It is a systemized approach that allows the practitioner to answer the question, "What purpose does this behavior serve?"

Prior to the development of a BIP, the team should develop an FBA. Although the FBA provides crucial information to guide the BIP, it is not required by law in this instance. Let us explain it another way: When a student's behavior impedes his or her learning or the learning of others, the IEP team will consider developing a BIP. The FBA is important to the BIP, but the IEP team is not required by federal law to complete an FBA prior to the development and subsequent implementation of a BIP.

So, is an FBA ever mandated by federal law? According to IDEA 2004, an FBA is required when a student with an IEP has a disciplinary change of placement for behavior that is determined to be a manifestation of the student's disability. Note the following regarding these actions (you can read more at http://idea.ed.gov):

"1.  *Consecutive suspensions past 10 days:* On the 11th day in a row, services must be provided and a manifestation determination is required. (Often a student will exceed 10 days awaiting expulsion proceedings.) If this misbehavior is determined to be a manifestation of his or her disability, an FBA is required; otherwise, it is not required following the manifestation determination.

2.  *Cumulative suspensions past 10 days in a school year:* The principal or other responsible person is required to determine if this series of removals constitutes a pattern resulting in a de facto *change in placement* because: 10 days were exceeded, this misconduct is substantially similar to previous behaviors and other factors such as length of each removal, proximity of removals, and total amount of time of cumulative removals suggests this suspension is subjecting the student to a change in placement. If it is concluded that this suspension does constitute a pattern (that is, a de facto change in placement), then a manifestation determination must be conducted. If the behavior is a manifestation of the student's disability, then an FBA must be conducted unless the school district had conducted an FBA before the behavior that resulted in the "change of placement" had occurred. They must then implement a behavior intervention plan for the student. If a behavior intervention plan already has been developed, the team must then review the behavior intervention plan, and modify it, as necessary, to address the problematic behavior."

In summary, IDEA 2004 mandates the implementation of an FBA when (1) a student has been suspended for past 10 consecutive days or past 10 cumulative days in a school year, and (2) the IEP team determines that the misbehavior in the past 10 consecutive days is a manifestation of the student's disability, or (3) the pattern of misconduct in the past 10 cumulative days constitutes a pattern that has essentially created a change of placement for the student. That resulting pattern is then determined to be a manifestation of the student's disability.

Although not legally required in every behavioral instance, IDEA 2004 does consider the use of an FBA as *best practice*. In education, *best practice* could be considered the consistent and effective implementation of successful methodologies. As a practitioner using protocols for behavior, using a protocol to fidelity is best practice. If a student is identified as having behaviors that might impede his or her learning or the learning of others, choosing to assess the student and implement effective behavioral change strategies is demonstrating best practices. Utilizing an FBA as an assessment tool in evaluation and developing a BIP would be deemed best practices.

Additionally, IDEA 2004 does not define the specific guidelines for the development of an FBA. Just as with the BIP, it is vague in the expectations for what an FBA will include. For this reason, the FBA may look very different from state to state, and even from district to district. Within the USA, states can differ significantly in the requirements regarding public education. Some states have chosen to impose greater regulations than those mandated by IDEA 2004 for their schools. In these states, they have outlined more specific requirements, content, and expectations of the FBA and BIP. Even in the area of legislation, each state chooses what they will require beyond the mandates found in IDEA 2004. An advantage to requiring or even legally mandating the use of an FBA or a BIP is that it helps to bring uniformity to the process in these regions. Without these requirements, the vagueness of IDEA 2004 language regarding the FBA and BIP leaves some areas open for interpretation. State-specific information regarding FBA and BIP requirements should be accessible through each state's Department of Education. If you work for a school system and need to clarify if your area has paperwork or forms that are required for an FBA or a BIP, you can contact your school district's Special Education Department to inquire. We have included contact information for your state's Department of Education and Office of Special Education in Appendix A.

## Strategy Two: Understand the Scope

As noted, FBA is not something that is used in just an experimental manner. FBA is an ongoing tool that is promoted across settings and even required by federal law within the school system. To utilize this tool, it is important to understand the terminology associated with FBA. So, let us widen the scope from the roots of the FBA to the actual meaning of the letters: *F—B—A*.

**Function**  The basic premise of creating an FBA is that through a series of methods, one can determine the relationship between two events: a behavior and a consequence (Iwata et al. 2000). When the impact is studied and understood, a functional relationship can be identified between the two. For instance, 5-year-old Alex is standing and screaming in front of the television. His father turns the channel to cartoons. Alex quits screaming. In this scenario, there is a functional relationship between Alex's screaming behavior and the television channel being changed to cartoons. In the future, when Alex wants to watch cartoons, it is likely that he will stand in front of the television and scream. If this scenario is repeated, the screaming behavior is reinforced. Thus, it becomes more likely that every time Alex wants to watch cartoons, he will display the screaming behavior.

However, the scenario could have been different. Alex wants to watch cartoons. He is screaming in front of the television. His father enters the room and attempts to get Alex to verbalize what he wants. It is unsuccessful and Alex continues to scream. At this point, Alex's father does not turn on the television. Instead, he sends Alex to his room. For Alex, the event is unsuccessful. His screaming behavior did not gain access to the cartoons he wanted to watch. Therefore, the screaming behavior would not have been reinforced. If this scenario is repeated, the screaming behavior would most likely decrease.

When determining the functional relationship between behavior and consequence, it is important to ascertain the impact the two have on each other. Understanding the degree of relationship allows the consequence to be manipulated successfully, thus allowing for impacting behavior change.

**Behavior**  As noted, there is an underlying assumption in behaviorism that all behavior is learned. This is an important foundational understanding. Without it, there would be no reason to conduct an FBA. Furthermore, any behavior can be assessed. In most instances, it is the interfering or negative behavior that seems to warrant assessment. One of the ways we have found to effectively teach behavior to practitioners is to start with our senses.

For a moment, listen carefully. What do you hear? Is it the sound of traffic? Is it a barking dog? Now, look up from this book. What do you see? Is it a computer screen? Is it your work desk? Think about what you have experienced over the past 2 h. What was that experience like? What is the world like around you? What do you see people doing? What do you hear people doing? How would you describe that to someone on the phone, or even in a different country?

- *What can be seen, heard, or experienced?* Behaviorism focuses on external factors. It is the way people act, behave, and react that can be studied, not what they think or feel. Therefore, the FBA approach focuses on external factors. Let us go back to Aaliyah. She is crying as the math assignment is handed out. A behavioral focus would be to observe the antecedent, behavior, and consequence. What is it that is seen? As for behavior, it is Aaliyah's crying. The tears are rolling down her cheeks. Let us look at Alex. Can we see screaming? No. Can we hear or experience screaming? Yes. Screaming is the behavior that Alex is exhibiting.
- *What cannot be seen, heard, or experienced?* The behavior to be addressed in the FBA will be seen, heard, or experienced. Although there are influences that might impact behavior that are internal, these influences are not behaviors. These influences might be a physical illness or a level of cognitive functioning. In an FBA, these will be considered, but not as behavior. In regard to behavior, the FBA will not focus on internal states, conditions, or moods. These cannot be seen. For those of you who might say, "Aha! We can see Aaliyah's mood. She is crying," let us clarify a little more. It is the *crying* you can see; it is not the mood. Perhaps if Aaliyah were to enter counseling, her therapist would identify some type of anxiety that is linked to math. Maybe Aaliyah would begin to process her feelings in regard to math and her crying episodes. It is possible this will be effective for Aaliyah. Yet, in compiling and quantifying data in the classroom, it is only what can be observed that is studied or gathered. And an FBA is a method to gather, compile, study, and subsequently alter behavior that can be seen.

**Assessment** FBA is an evaluative process with an intended outcome. The outcome is a hypothesis that reports the functional relationship between behavior and consequence. The implication of this hypothesis will allow for variables to be manipulated and supports to be implemented to maintain, increase, or decrease behavior (Jolivette et al. 2000). Within this process, there are also methods that will be used to gather, study, and compile the behavioral data. These include records reviews, direct observations, interviews, inventories, evaluations, and questionnaires. The compilation of this entire process manifests itself in the form of an FBA.

# Strategy Three: What to Do

Throughout this book, there will be guidance on how to write an FBA. Prior to delving into each area, we are going to sharpen your vocabulary by introducing you to or reminding you about the language used in the FBA approach. We also want to highlight areas that you will focus on during this process. To underscore some of these points, we are introducing them to you now:

1. *Respondent*—For the purposes of this section, let us consider the subject a *respondent*. For instance, Aaliyah or Alex would be the individual whose behavior has become problematic. In considering the respondent, there are numerous factors that impact behavior. Although we might not be attempting to change these factors, they will need to be considered nonetheless.
   - Physiological—Does the respondent have mental health issues, illness, genetic disorders, chronic conditions, other types of impairments or difficulties that are impacting the targeted behavior?
   - Cultural—Are there different social, responsive, behavioral, or influential differences between the respondent and the environment in which the targeted behavior is occurring?
   - Pharmacological—Is the respondent prescribed medication or treatment that is impacting the targeted behavior?

2. *Distant setting events*—This might be a new phrase to your vocabulary. If so, a distant setting event is an unexpected or unique situation that helps to increase or decrease the likelihood of a behavior. These events do not happen immediately before the behavior occurs (such as an antecedent). Rather, they are distant (such as the morning or evening before), or they can be ongoing. These events are sometimes called slow triggers, noted for their lack of immediacy when impacting behavior. Although slow or distant, these setting events still impact the behavioral responses of the respondent. Here are some of those events:
   - *Life events*—Has something significant happened that impacts the respondent's behavior, such as a death, traumatic event, etc.?
   - *Disruptive events*—Has something changed in the respondent's routine? Did the respondent miss the bus? Is it the respondent's birthday? Did the respondent's dog run away the night before?
   - *Physiological events*—Is the respondent sick? Is the respondent hurting or aching from an event, such as falling down?

3. *Context*—The context is the circumstances in which the behavior occurs.
   - *Where?* Setting—inside classroom, playground, office, cafeteria, hallway
   - *Who?* People present—peers, teachers, parents, administrative staff, paraprofessionals
   - *When?* Time of day—morning, afternoon, a specific time, a specific season
   - *What?* Events/occurrence factors—curriculum, actions (test being returned, transitioning, given a directive, etc.)

4. *Three-term contingency* (stimulus-response-stimulus)—Developed from the work of B. F. Skinner, the three-term contingency is also referred to as the ABCs of behavior. This model explains how the environment elicits behavior and how the consequences of behavior can affect the future occurrence of behavior.
5. *Antecedent*—This is the preceding stimulus. It is the event, experience, or circumstance that happened just before the behavior. (It will involve some or all of the variables listed under context.) For example, Aaliyah's teacher, Ms. Mealer, hands out the math assignment.
6. *Consequence*—This is the event, experience, or circumstance that happened right after the behavior (reinforcers or punishers). Aaliyah's teacher, Ms. Mealer, comforts Aaliyah and helps her answer the first few questions.
7. *Function*—The function of the behavior is what purpose it serves the respondent. We have seen this presented many different ways. Primarily, the function of the behavior has one of the following purposes:
   - *To gain/obtain*
   - *To avoid/escape*

We are going to expand on that in this book. We are going to further include the following purposes:

   - *To access*
   - *To communicate*

What is the respondent trying to access, avoid/escape, communicate, or gain/obtain?


## Strategy Four: Application

The following should be considered a brief overview of the steps that will be explained in detail throughout this book. One difficulty that you might find within the public school system is the lack of uniformity in procedural expectations regarding the FBA process. We realize that there will be many instances when you will be mandated to use a specific format or meet a procedural demand. In light of this, here are the steps that we feel best sum up this process.

*Who should conduct FBA?* There are two ways to conduct an FBA: a team approach or a specialist approach.

- The team approach is a collaborative effort among individuals working directly with the student or client.
- A specialist approach would be conducted by a professional within an area of specialization, such as a psychologist, school psychologist, behavior analyst, behavior specialist, or behavior counselor. This approach would still entail the involvement of those working directly with the student, but would be mostly limited to providing the specialist with collected data, history and information, and interviews.

*What is the systematic process for developing an FBA?*

## *Process*

1. Identify target behaviors
2. Identify the context in which the behaviors occur
3. Collect data on the respondent (indirect and direct)

## *Purpose*

4. Analyze the data
5. Develop a hypothesis (function)

*What happens after the FBA is completed?*

## *Planning*

6. Implement an intervention plan (replacement behaviors, supports, interventions, and strategies)
7. Evaluate the progress of the respondent

## *Prevention*

8. Create a climate, culture, and community where prevention is possible
9. Change plan as needed

## Strategy 5: What *Not* to Do

When writing an FBA, here are a few things you do *not* want to do.

- *Skip a step*—Each step of the development is important. Missing a step will impact the reliability and validity of the FBA.
- *Forget the parental consent*—If you work in the school setting, the FBA is an evaluation. Therefore, to complete one, you need parental consent.
- *Ignore state and federal regulations*—Be sure to check with your state to determine the most current rules and regulations regarding implementing an FBA. You can access federal regulations for the IDEA 2004 at http://idea.ed.gov/.

- *Report inaccurate information*—Whenever observing a student or interviewing an involved individual, be sure to provide accurate and objective information.

## A Before-You-Proceed Checklist

1. Understand the parameters that define behavior.
2. Understand the applications for the words function, behavior, and assessment.
3. Know the definitions for the following words or phrases: distant setting events, context, antecedent, and consequence.
4. Recognize that the function of a behavior serves to access, avoid/escape, communicate, or gain/obtain.

**Author Takeaways**

*Takeaway from Stephanie, the behavior specialist:*

It is important to remember that a recurring problematic behavior is rarely isolated to one instance or factor. Identifying the contextual elements that impact behavior is not only important but also necessary to impact behavioral change. This process takes more than just one observation. It requires the assessor to gather and examine data from many sources. Accuracy and effectiveness is built on objectivity and multiple sources of information. The FBA will be compromised when building on solitary sources and opinions only.

*Takeaway from Alan, the school psychologist:*

An FBA is a process—it is not something that you are going to learn right away and complete quickly. It takes a great deal of preparation to get ready for an FBA, and it takes strong insight and analytical skills in order to make sense of the data. When doing an FBA, take into consideration the time commitment needed for this process. School psychologists conducting FBAs must also consider their testing workload, meetings they have scheduled, and consultation commitments.

## References

Becker, S. P., Paternite, C. E., Evans, S. W., Andrews, C., Christensen, O. A., Kraan, E. M., & Weist, M. D. (2011). Eligibility, assessment, and educational placement issues for students classified with emotional disturbance: Federal and state-level analyses. *School Mental Health, 3*(1), 24–34.

Bradley, R., Doolittle, J., & Bartolotta, R. (2008). Building on the data and adding to the discussion: The experiences and outcomes of students with emotional disturbance. *Journal of Behavioral Education, 17*(1), 4–23.

Dixon, D. R., Vogel, T., & Tarbox, J. (2012). A brief history of functional analysis and applied behavior analysis. In J. L. Matson (Ed.), *Functional assessment for challenging behaviors* (pp. 3–24). New York: Springer.

Iwata, B. A., Dorsey, M. F., Slifer, K. J., Bauman, K. E., & Richman, G. S. (1982). Toward a functional analysis of self-injury. *Analysis and Intervention in Developmental Disabilities, 2*(1), 3–20.

Iwata, B. A., Wallace, M. D., Kahng, S. W., Lindber, J. S., Roscoe, E. M., Conners, J., et al. (2000). Skill acquisition in the implementation of functional analysis methodology. *Journal of Applied Behavior Analysis, 33,* 181–194.

Jolivette, K., Scott, T. M., & Nelson, C. M. (2000). The link between functional behavior assessments (FBAs) and behavioral intervention plans (BIPs). *ERIC Digest*, E592, EDO-00-1.

Pavlov, I. V. (1927). *Conditioned reflexes: An investigation of the physiological activity of the cerebral cortex.* London: Oxford University Press.

Sanford, C., Newman, L., Wagner, M., Cameto, R., Knokey, A.-M., & Shaver, D. (2011). *The post-high school outcomes of young adults with disabilities up to 6 years after high school: Key findings from the national longitudinal transition study-2 (NLTS2) (NCSER 2011–3004).* Menlo Park: SRI International.

Skinner, B. F. (1953). *Science and human behavior.* New York: The Free Press.

Smith, C. R., Katsiyannis, A., & Ryan, J. B. (2011). Challenges of serving students with emotional and behavioral disorders: Legal and policy considerations. *Behavioral Disorders, 36*(3), 185–194.

Thorndike, E. L. (1911). *Animal intelligence.* New York: Macmillan.

Watson, J. B. (1913). Psychology as the behaviorist views it. *Psychological Review, 20,* 158–177.

Wilmshurst, L., & Brue, A. W. (2010). *The complete guide to special education: Expert advice on evaluations, IEPs, and helping kids succeed* (2nd ed.). San Francisco: Jossey-Bass.

# Part II
# Phase I: Process

*Process* is the beginning phase of functional behavioral assessment.

**Professional Responsibilities** Within *Process*, the practitioner would make preparations, review records, interview the student and other contributing parties, utilize assessments, collect data, and complete observations.

**Alternative View** The *Process* phase could also be considered the *doing* or *working* phase. This phase is about gathering, asking, reviewing, and observing.

**Task List**

1. Gather team
2. Define target behavior(s)
3. Assign team responsibilities or contact specialist

The following tasks will be completed by the practitioner or a team member:

4. Review records
5. Interviews
6. Distribute and gather questionnaires
7. Observe subject

**Goal** By the end of this phase, the practitioner would have gathered accurate and reliable data on the target behavior.

# Chapter 3
# Process: Preparing for the Functional Behavioral Assessment

## What You Need to Know

Benjamin Franklin is quoted as saying: "By failing to prepare, you are preparing to fail." As we begin this chapter on preparation, we are actually beginning the first phase of our multiphasic approach to the development of a functional behavioral assessment (FBA). *Process* is the starting phase and is identifiable by characteristics of gathering, collecting, asking, and reviewing. We have encouraged you to view the progression of this group of methods as steps taking you closer to an informational result.

We enter the Process phase stressing Mr. Franklin's fundamental philosophy. Careful preparation will be a key element to the success of an FBA. There are many stages throughout each phase in this approach. It will be difficult to execute these stages without forethought to actionable planning. The most effective FBAs are often built with accurate data collecting, objective observations of the student, informative parent, staff and student interviews, insightful questionnaires and surveys, and a thorough review of the child's history and records. Too often, we have encountered practitioners attempting to back track and complete an interview, record review, or observation that they simply forgot. Spending time preparing helps to avoid the missteps that not only increase momentary stressors but also increase the likelihood of missing valuable data. Skipping this step can impact the overall efficacy of the FBA process.

## Strategy One: Understand the Basics

As we noted in Chap. 1, we have included a case snapshot to act as a guide and perhaps interject some levity within the book. The culmination of these vignettes will be a completed FBA and behavior intervention plan found in Chap. 12. Here, we would like to introduce you to Willow Wilding, a second-grade student and a budding artist.

© Springer International Publishing Switzerland 2016        25
S. M. Hadaway, A. W. Brue, *Practitioner's Guide to Functional Behavioral Assessment,*
Autism and Child Psychopathology Series, DOI 10.1007/978-3-319-23721-3_3

For a moment, we will consider that you have been working as a special education teacher at Good Hope Elementary School. In one classroom you support, you have a second-grade student whose behaviors are becoming increasingly disruptive in the classroom. Willow Wilding's behaviors are interfering, and both you and the general education teacher are spending important teaching time chasing her around the room. By the end of the day, the classroom floor is littered with torn papers, turned over desks and items ripped from the walls. Mostly, this catastrophic mess is due to Willow's antics. She is chaotic and disruptive. Worse yet, other students are beginning to follow her lead. Mrs. Huffing, the general education teacher, is quickly growing tired of replacing word walls and bulletin board items. She has already begun to talk about more service time for the student. You have tried stickers and verbal praise. You have introduced a token economy. You have even attempted to teach her a happy dance you learned from watching YouTube. You have taken away recess and contacted her mother, but nothing you have tried has seemed to work. Despite your best efforts, the behavior has persisted and you are at a loss. Unfortunately, it is only the fifth day of school and you are already exhausted. In a moment of opportunity, you literally chase down the behavior interventionist, Donny Data, and beg him for help.

He asks, "Have you attempted or has a functional behavioral assessment been completed in the past?" You weakly smile, "Ummmm."

Certainly, preparation begins with identifying the student who actually needs an FBA. No doubt, you might be able to think of more than one. But, how do you know that the student you have in mind is a good candidate? Let us answer the most basic question first.

## *Who Should Have a Functional Behavioral Assessment?*

If an individual is exhibiting behaviors that are interfering with learning, an FBA is certainly a viable option. As noted by Severson et al. (2007), schools face increased pressure to be more proactive and to address the needs of students who demonstrate problematic behaviors in the classroom. If the behavior is significantly atypical, disruptive, and/or inappropriate in the environment, an FBA can be completed on their behavior.

## *Should Only Children or Adolescents Have a Functional Behavioral Assessment?*

No. There are many adults in residential, treatment, and/or community programs that would benefit from the FBA.

## *In a School Setting, Can Only Students Receiving Special Educational Services Have a Functional Behavioral Assessment?*

Within the school system, a student eligible for services due to an identified disability will have an individualized education program (Wilmshurst and Brue 2010). The student's team, comprising the student's parents, teachers, and other identified support personnel, will have developed the Individualized Education Program (IEP). If a student receiving exceptional educational services has behaviors that impede his or her learning, the team will consider developing a behavior intervention plan. Prior to the behavior intervention plan, an FBA should be developed. If you recall, this is considered best practices by federal law. The information gained from the FBA will guide the behavior intervention plan.

However, let us not make an assumption that only students identified as eligible for special education have interfering behaviors. Speaking from our collective experiences, this would be a fallible assumption to make. Students who might need an FBA are not limited to students supported through exceptional education. General education students might also demonstrate interfering behaviors as well. In the past, the FBA process has generally been utilized with students receiving special education services or who have been referred for evaluation (Quinn et al. 2001). However, there is an ever-broadening area of research addressing the FBA and students not identified as having disabilities. Moreno and Bullock (2011) report that the use of the FBA is becoming more accepted throughout all populations, including assisting non-disabled students exhibiting interfering behaviors in the general educational setting.

Let us go back to Good Hope Elementary. You are talking with the behavior interventionist:

> You weakly manage to ask, "Functional behavioral assessment? I'm not sure. If she doesn't, um, how do I proceed with all of that?"
> "Well," Donny Data queries. "Is she receiving special education services? If so, are you her case manager? All of this information should be in her file. You have looked, haven't you?" You bite your lip. You have looked, but you just don't remember. After all, it is the first week of school and you can't even remember all the last names of your students yet!

## *If All of This Begins by Identifying the Student, What Comes Next?*

There has to be someone who initiates this process. If a student receives special education services, it is our opinion that this person would naturally be the case manager. It would be the person responsible for overseeing the legal mandates regarding the student's education. Another great idea is to have the team designate a team coordinator. This does not mean the case manager or team coordinator is responsible for executing each step of the FBA process; rather, this individual gathers together the individuals necessary for the development of the FBA, oversees data collection, communicates with other team members, and facilitates the FBA process (Neitzel and Bogin 2008). If a student does not receive special education supports, this person would most likely be the student's homeroom teacher or teacher of record, school counselor, or school social worker. For individuals in residential, treatment, or community programs requiring the FBA, this would be the individual who gathers the treatment team or manages the resident's supports.

Combined, we have about 30 years of experience actually working within the public education system. Additionally, we have worked beyond the school system in universities and community programs supporting populations with diverse needs including mental illness, severe, emotional disorders, addictive behaviors, and cognitive delays. We have served in professional capacities, such as board members and community liaisons. In our experiences, environments tend to handle behavioral challenges in two ways, specifically when writing behavior intervention plans and FBAs. To define these clearly for practitioners, we identify these problem-solving methods as approaches. In our opinion, these approaches are typically the team approach and the specialist approach. (This is another chance to test your knowledge from Chap. 2.) Within this two-armed paradigm, organizations vary in their rigidity to these approaches. Some have clearly defined rules and others handle the matter more loosely. Despite their varying levels of strict adherence to a selection process, in our opinion the determinants for choosing an approach seems to be the practices and policies developed by the residential program, treatment center, or school district in which the individual is supported; the severity of behavior the individual is exhibiting; access to a wide range of professional personnel; and access to funding.

In a moment, we will be discussing the conditional expectations that define the two approaches, team or specialist. At some point, you or your organization will make the decision as to which approach to use. As part of that decision-making process, we would like to offer you our thoughts on this matter.

In 2014, we began contemplating writing this book. Since a significant portion of our work life is spent within the public education system, we know the types of responsibilities that individuals are asked to undertake with sometimes limited training. For many years, we have been concerned about the efficacy of behavior planning, especially with the use of the FBA. Since the FBA originates from the well-controlled world of experimental research, it should be noted that there have been professional concerns expressed that the reliability and validity of methods employed in the FBA process cannot be adequately replicated in a less-controlled environment, such as a school. A range of concerns has been cited, including the difficulty in training staff to execute the method adequately (McIntosh and Av-Gay 2007). In research conducted by Benazzi et al. (2006), there were three conditions identified, which met the criteria for an appropriate amount of technical adequacy (understanding and executing behavioral knowledge and techniques) and contextual fit (a plan designed to be effective within the specific learning environment). These conditions were noted as: "(a) knowledge about the student, (b) knowledge about the context, and (c) knowledge about behavioral theory." Other authors have noted that certain strategies have been helpful in promoting desired behavior in students, including high teacher expectations (Marzano 2010; McKown and Weinstein 2008), motivating instructions with a high level of student engagement (Emmer and Stough 2001; Sutherland and Wehby 2001), clearly stated rules (Kerr and Nelson 2006; Sprick and Daniels 2010; Tanol et al. 2010), established routines and procedures (Evertson et al. 2006), good teacher–student rapport (Marzano 2003), and efficient use of time each school day (Lee 2006).

Going forward, we strongly advocate that the conditions identified by Benazzi et al. (2006) are part of your decision-making process. It is important to have participants, team members, or contributing informants in either approach who know the student, know what will work in the environment, and have knowledge of behavioral theory.

With that in mind, let us take a closer look at these two approaches.

**The Team Approach** Within a collaborative environment, the FBA is perhaps more commonly developed within a team atmosphere. A student or resident's team will consist of the people who support the individual while they are participating in the educational program, community program, or treatment program. This might include family members, teachers, case managers, social workers, counselors, job coaches, advocates, speech therapists, occupational therapists, physical therapists, and art therapists. It might also include additional members with a specific insight into the behavioral challenges, medical conditions, or educational curriculum related to the individual's needs, such as psychiatrists, school psychologists, clinical psychologists, doctors, autism specialists, curriculum interventionists, behavior specialists, and behavior analysts.

**The Specialist Approach** In certain schools, residential programs, or community programs, there might be a specialist who has been procured to write all the FBAs. This person is typically employed by your organization and is the "go-to person" when a resident or student is exhibiting significant behavioral challenges. If that is the case in your program or school, this individual might be a school psychologist, behavior specialist, behavior interventionist, behavior analyst, or autism specialist.

For some organizations, it is not feasible to employ a specialist full-time or even part-time. In these cases, the organization might contract services as needed. Even though the organization has well-trained staff, such as special education teachers or counselors, there might be specific conditions when an outside specialist is contracted to provide a more extensive assessment.

Whether the specialist is employed full-time, part-time, or contracted for the organization, typically his or her services are requested when an individual's behavior has become dangerous or highly interfering, the situation surrounding the behavior has become complicated, or the relationship between the program and family has become adversarial. A specialist will have expertise in a behavioral area and offer insight that other professionals might not possess. Also, the specialist is often a neutral party that might be necessary if trust has been broken between the family and the program. In the past, we have noticed that there are programs that secure the services of a specialist with ease. We have also seen this process become unnecessarily complicated. Much of this hinges on clear, definable protocols.

In order to gain access to a specialist within your system or procure the services of a specialist outside of your organization, there should a clear set of steps to guide this process. If the specialist is from within your organization, the protocol would most likely be a referral process. If the program is part of the school system, the referral should begin with gaining written parental consent for an evaluation. Once that is gained, a referral should be sent to the specialist. A comprehensive referral would include the contact information of the individual, information on the classroom or program the student is currently attending, background information including medications, diagnosis and identified eligibility for current programming, target behavior(s) with clear and definable definitions, situations in which the target behavior(s) occurs, methods and strategies that have been attempted, case manager contact information, and any other information that might appear relevant, such as a recent life change. Community, residential, or treatment programs might have a referral process similar to this. Depending on the age and condition of the individual, consent might be given by the individual or needed from a guardian or parent. If the specialist is outside of your organization, it is imperative that confidentiality is considered. You must gain parental or individual consent to share information and secure the specialist. Additionally, your organization will have to secure funding to pay for the outside specialist's services. Therefore, some type of approval for physical entry into the program and payment of services will have to be secured. Along with this, the outside specialist will need access to the same type of information that would be provided to a specialist within your organization. This would include all the information that was included in the referral packet. One further note, even if a specialist develops the FBA, the input of the team is still valuable. Information gathered from those involved in the individual's life gives critical data to the specialist. There is never a time when an FBA is completed without some form of input from the team.

Of course, understanding the differences between these two approaches is great, but it does not change one important point. Whether your organization uses the team approach or the specialist approach, there still must be *one person* who begins this process. The team coordinator or case manager is the contact person throughout all phases of FBA development—*Process, Purpose, Planning, and Prevention*. Without the case manager or team coordinator, this process would come to an abrupt halt.

> Think back to your situation at Good Hope Elementary School. If you remember, the behavior interventionist has asked about the student's IEP. As you stand there biting your lip and feeling lost, you make a decision.
> "You know, I probably need to look through her chart one more time." You head off to find out if your student has a functional behavioral assessment.

## Strategy Two: Understand the Scope

> As it turns out, Willow Wilding does not have an FBA. It is now the third week of school and you are trying to organize a meeting to discuss her behavior. You know that the general education teacher, Priscilla Huffing, needs to be invited. Mr. and Mrs. Wilding also must have an invitation. The speech language pathologist and the occupational therapist need an invitation. Donny Data, the behavior interventionist, is definitely getting an invitation. But who else? And, how are you supposed to lead a meeting when you just aren't even that sure about what an FBA actually is?

Whether a team approach or a specialist approach is used, there will be certain individuals necessary for the completion of a successful FBA. These team members each possess unique experiences and insights regarding the student.

## *So Who Are the Team Members?*

Any staff member who works directly with the individual is a team member. The team might also include specialists within the environment who might provide additional insight and information into the FBA process. This could include doctors, guidance counselors, therapists, school psychologists, social workers, autism specialists, and behavior specialists, to name a few. Even if you are using the team approach, specialists can help to guide and consult with the team about behavior.

## *What if the Individual Is Doing Well with One Staff Member—Should that Staff Member Still Be Included?*

Yes, it is important to have everyone's input. If the individual does not exhibit behaviors with one or more staff members, those staff members might be able to provide valuable insight into the triggers, needs, and preferences of the individual. When a behavior does not occur it is often just as illuminating as when it does occur.

## *Is the Parent a Team Member?*

If a student is eligible for special education, then the parent, legal guardian, or legal caregiver is a member of the IEP team. If the student is in the general population, the parent is also a team member.

## *What Is a Parent's Role as a Team Member?*

Certainly, the parent must give their consent for the student to receive an FBA. In a question-and-answer session by the Office of Special Education and Rehabilitative Services (OSERS) regarding IDEA 2004, OSERS further clarifies their position on the FBA. Given below are the questions and answers from their Web site (http://www2.ed.gov/about/offices/list/osers/index.html)

> *Question E-4:* Is consent required to do an FBA for a child?
> *Answer:* Yes. An FBA is generally understood to be an individualized evaluation of a child in accordance with 34 CFR §§ 300.301 through 300.311 to assist in determining whether the child is, or continues to be, a child with a disability. The FBA process is frequently used to determine the nature and extent of the special education and related services that the child needs, including the need for a BIP. As with other individualized evaluation procedures, and consistent with 34 CFR § 300.300(a) and (c), parental consent is required for an FBA to be conducted as part of the initial evaluation or a reevaluation.

Since the FBA is evaluative in nature, parental consent is required prior to conducting an FBA for both students receiving special education supports and students receiving the general education curriculum. You might be thinking: "We do not require parents to give consent for every evaluation we do. Every week there is a reading and math test. We certainly don't have written consent for those measures." If an evaluation is given to every student in the classroom, it is not individualized. It is unnecessary to gain consent for what could be considered typical or common. The Office of Special Education Programs (OSEP) responds to an inquiry from Glenna Gallo on April 2, 2013, clarifying that parental consent must be gained for an FBA if it is individualized (see https://www2.ed.gov/policy/speced/guid/idea/memosdcltrs/acc-12-017845r-ut-gallo-fba-4-2-13.pdf). If it were to be used for an entire classroom as part of a classroom management program, then consent would not need to be gained. In that scenario, all students would receive the FBA. Without parental consent, the FBA cannot be conducted for an individualized purpose.

The parent remains involved in the FBA process after parental consent is gained. The staff will be responsible for gathering data, conducting interviews, and developing the FBA. The parent is involved in this process through the parent interview conducted by a school staff member and subsequently in the meeting where the FBA is reported to them and a behavior intervention plan is developed. As part of the student's team, the parent will actively contribute to identifying strategies, interventions, reinforcers, and any other discussion regarding behavioral planning. This helps to decrease the burden on teachers, who are sometimes faced with developing and implementing a behavior intervention plan without assistance (Losinski et al. 2015).

## What Is a Staff Member's Role as a Team Member?

Any team member has the same responsibility. Show up and be prepared. In a collaborative environment, a team member might help with the development of an FBA by participating in interviews, conducting interviews, gathering data, and reviewing records and observations. A staff member should also be prepared to discuss, listen, reflect, and help develop the interventions and strategies that will be used in behavior planning. Perhaps not required, but certainly very helpful is to maintain a positive attitude throughout the process.

## Strategy Three: What to Do

So, the day is fast approaching for Willow Wilding's meeting. You understand the role of each team member. You want to have a good meeting. You spot your lead special education teacher as she is headed to her car a few days before the meeting. She doesn't look happy when you prevent her from leaving.

You speak quickly. "Gwen, I hate to catch you as you are going home." You notice that she rolls her eyes.

"What is it now?"

"Well, about this FBA meeting. I've invited everyone, but I'm not really sure how to conduct this meeting. Can you help me out?"

She sighs noticeably. "Email me your schedule for tomorrow and I'll squeeze you in between meetings."

You nod and she's out of the parking lot before you can get in another word! You can hear her tires squealing all the way to the road!

## What Am I Supposed to Do?

So, you are the case manager or team coordinator for a student whose behavior is escalating. There are multiple ways to complete an FBA. It has been our experience that two to four meetings might be necessary for the FBA process to be complete. It is probably best to plan for a minimum of two meetings.

## But, What Am I Supposed to Do?

At your first meeting, be prepared to discuss student behavior, past strategies, new strategies, and the possibility of developing an FBA. It should not be assumed that an FBA will be developed. It is the team's responsibility to determine a course of action. You should lead the team in a discussion about the behavior. If the team determines that FBA is the best option, discuss the need for consent. The parent or legal guardian has a right to deny the assessment. If the parent or legal guardian is willing for the student to be assessed, then they should sign a form to consent to the evaluation. Your district will have this form available for you.

A central component of the meeting will be the data that have already been gathered. All team members should bring their behavioral data to the meeting. With this data, the team will work to develop one to three target behaviors to be assessed. The target behaviors will be clearly defined. If sufficient data are presented regarding the target behaviors, the team could perhaps determine the baseline for them. Even though the team has an idea of the behaviors, they are not clearly defined until the meeting. Therefore, it is improbable that the team would have collected sufficient data on unidentified target behavior(s). If the team were to have sufficient data, they could go forward with assigning responsibilities and setting a timeline for developing the FBA. If a specialist approach is used, then the team should also complete the referral form for the specialist.

In the event that the team does not have baseline data on the target behaviors, there should be a second meeting. The second meeting should be used to review the target behaviors and present the baseline data on the target behaviors. The team will then assign responsibilities. These will include questionnaires, interviews, review of student records (which should have already been done), observations, and determination of the length of time until the information will be assembled.

We do want to make it clear that target behaviors can be modified or changed based on descriptive analysis and data gathered from interviews. Sometimes when a specialist is brought in, the specialist might also redefine the target behaviors more clearly. We will talk more about target behaviors in Chap. 4. However, we want to remind you that this is a fluid process, and the introduction of additional information might prompt the team or specialist to modify or actually select new target behaviors.

During the third meeting, the team will take the information gathered and determine the function of the student's behavior. If a specialist approach has been used, the specialist will deliver the results of the FBA to the team.

## Strategy Four: Application

### Prior to the Meeting

*Step One* Gather student records. You want to have a good understanding of the child's history including social, academic, behavioral, emotional, cultural, familial, and physiological aspects. Consider these records:

- Individualized Education Program (IEP)
- Behavior intervention plan
- Disciplinary reports
- Historical information
- Attendance reports
- Assessment records
- 504 Plan
- RTI (response to intervention) records

*Step Two* Contact team members including the parent or legal caregiver with information regarding:

- Meeting date and time
- Data needed—this should include information on student's behavior and strategies that have been attempted

*Step Three* Gather the necessary paperwork—sign-in sheets, parental rights, parental consent form, referral form, any data collected on the student that is pertinent, and any paperwork designated by your district or state.

### During the Meeting

*Step Four* Present the current behavior difficulties or disciplinary event that prompted the meeting.

*Step Five* Review student records. Be sure to incorporate all the information that is relevant based on your pre-meeting review. If a student has a behavior intervention plan, this should be reviewed as well.

*Step Six* Facilitate a discussion on the student's overall functioning. Have team members discuss data, interventions, and how the student has progressed. Make sure to note the context in which the student does and does not exhibit problems. Include who is present, where it occurs, time of day, surrounding events, and any other relevant data.

*Step Seven* Determine a plan. If the team agrees to go forward with an FBA, be sure to know the policies and procedures your state and district have developed. If a specialist typically develops the FBA, gain parental consent, complete the referral papers, and submit them to the appropriate personnel. If team members typically develop the FBA, then gain parental consent.

*Step Eight* Identify target behavior(s). These are the impacting behaviors that most need to improve for the student to be successful. The team should operationalize these behaviors by making them measurable. A student can have one target behavior. If there are multiple behaviors, narrow them down to three.

*Step Nine* Present baseline data if available. If not, set a new meeting date to present baseline data.

*Step Ten* Assign responsibilities to each staff member.

- Parent interview
- Student interview
- Staff interview (this can be done at the time of meeting)
- Review history and student records (disciplinary reports, student support team folder, 504 Plan, response to intervention records, eligibility reports, IEP)
- Observations
- Additional assessments, informal inventories, surveys, or questionnaires

*Step Eleven* Set a date to reconvene and finalize the FBA.

In actuality, the team coordinator or case manager might be the one responsible for most of these duties. For instance, interviews have less variability when the same person does the interviewing. If you are primarily responsible for all the steps, make certain to consult with the school psychologist, behavior interventionist, or lead special education teacher along the way.

## Strategy Five: What Not to Do

As noted previously, the FBA requires the input of all team members. Gathering together members who will contribute to this process is important. No one can do this alone. Make certain to plan ahead. By having all the necessary paperwork, contributing team members, historical data, baseline data, and the current behavior intervention plan available at the time of the meeting, you will save yourself and the team some time. Most importantly, the team will be able to work toward providing the most effective interventions for the student in a timely manner. A week or two can make a significant difference in a student's or resident's life.

> Willow Wilding's meeting is tomorrow. Gwen has helped you with a plan. You feel good about it, but you run into Mr. Data in the hallway.
> "I wanted you to know that I may be running late for Willow's meeting tomorrow. Do you even know how to write a target behavior? If not, do you have time for me to go over a few basics now?"
> "Um...." you manage to get out. But, you think, "OH NO!!!"

## A Before-You-Proceed Checklist

1. Understand the difference between the team approach and the specialist approach.
2. Identify individuals who are part of the student's or the resident's team.
3. Familiarize yourself with the OSER guidelines on an FBA.
4. Familiarize yourself with the steps involved in an FBA meeting.

**Authors' Takeaways**

*Takeaway from Stephanie, the behavior specialist:*

Data: Even though you are just preparing to begin an FBA, data should already have been collected. Chances are this is not the first issue the student has had. In fact, the student might already have a behavior intervention plan in place. The data collected on that plan will be helpful in building further strategies and interventions to better support the student. Do not miss an opportunity to gather data, even when a student is not misbehaving in a classroom. It is also the exceptions that yield crucial information and can serve the team in developing an effective plan. Every team member can come to the table with data. Prior to the meeting, it is important that you gather some of this information. By analyzing it before the meeting, you can present data in the first meeting. Either way, the FBA is data driven. It is based not on opinions, but instead on analysis generated by the data.

*Takeaway from Alan, the school psychologist:*

As we mentioned early in the chapter, preparation is key to a successful FBA. Things can get offtrack quickly if you do not have all of the parts needed to make the FBA successful. Much of what you will need takes time to gather and a bit of research on your end. The time investment will be worth it, since the more information you have the more likely you may be to complete a thorough FBA. This is not the time for shortcuts; an individual's potential progress can hinge on the FBA, which will then lead to a behavior intervention plan.

# References

Benazzi, L. R., Horner, R. H., & Good, R. H. (2006). Effects of behavior support team composition on the technical adequacy and contextual fit of behavior support plans. *Journal of Special Education, 40*(3), 160–170.

Emmer, E. T., & Stough, L. M. (2001). Classroom management: A critical part of educational psychology, with implications for teacher education. *Educational Psychologist, 36*(2), 103–112.

Evertson, C. M., Emmer, E. T., & Worsham, M. E. (2006). *Classroom management for elementary teachers* (7th ed.). Boston: Pearson Allyn & Bacon.

Kerr, M. M., & Nelson, C. M. (2006). *Strategies for addressing behavior problems in the classroom* (5th ed.). Columbus: Merrill Prentice Hall.

Lee, D. L. (2006). Facilitating transitions between and within academic tasks. *Remedial and Special Education, 27*(5), 312–317.

Losinski, M., Maag, J. W., Katsiyannis, A., & Ryan, J. B. (2015). The use of structural behavioral assessment to develop interventions for secondary students exhibiting challenging behaviors. *Education and Treatment of Children, 38*(2), 149–174.

Marzano, R. (2010). High expectations for all. *Educational Leadership, 68*(1), 82–84.

Marzano, R. J., & Marzano, J. S. (2003). The key to classroom management. *Educational Leadership, 61*(1), 6–13.

McIntosh, K., & Av-Gay, H. (2007). Implications of current research on the use of functional behavior assessment and behavior support planning in school systems. *International Journal of Behavioral Consultation and Therapy, 3*(1), 38–52.

McKown, C., & Weinstein, R. (2008). Teacher expectations, classroom context, and the achievement gap. *Journal of School Psychology, 46*(3), 235–261.

Moreno, G., & Bullock, L. M. (2011). Principles of positive behaviour supports: Using the FBA as a problem-solving approach to address challenging behaviours beyond special populations. *Emotional and Behavioural Difficulties, 16*(2), 117–127.

Neitzel, J., & Bogin, J. (2008). *Steps for implementation: Functional behavior assessment*. Chapel Hill: The National Professional Development Center on Autism Spectrum Disorders, Frank Porter Graham Child Development Institute, The University of North Carolina.

Quinn, M. M., Gable, R. A., Fox, J., Rutherford, R. B., Acker, R. V., & Conroy, M. (2001). Putting quality functional assessment into practice in schools: A research agenda on behalf of E/BD students. *Education and Treatment of Children, 24*(3), 261–275.

Severson, H. H., Walker, H. M., Hope-Doolittle, J., Kratochwill, T. R., & Gresham, F. M. (2007). Proactive, early screening to detect behaviorally at-risk students: Issues, approaches, emerging innovations, and professional practices. *Journal of School Psychology, 45*(2), 193–223.

Sprick, R., & Daniels, K. (2010). Managing student behavior. *Principal Leadership, 11*(1), 18–21.

Sutherland, K. S., & Wehby, J. H. (2001). Exploring the relationship between increased opportunities to respond to academic requests and the academic and behavioral outcomes of students with EBD: A review. *Remedial and Special Education, 22*, 113–121.

Tanol, G., Johnson, L., McComas, J., & Cote, E. (2010). Responding to rule violations or rule following: A comparison of two versions of the Good Behavior Game with kindergarten students. *Journal of School Psychology, 48*(6), 337–355.

Wilmshurst, L., & Brue, A. W. (2010). *The complete guide to special education: Expert advice on evaluations, IEPs, and helping kids succeed* (2nd ed.). San Francisco: Jossey-Bass.

# Chapter 4
# Process: Identifying Target Behaviors

## What You Need to Know

Preparation has opened the door for the working phase of functional behavioral assessment (FBA). An FBA will be used to assess a wide range of challenging behaviors in individuals who do and do not have a particular disability (Losinski et al. 2015). The target behavior is the focal point of an FBA, both literally and figuratively. It is the behavior that will be reviewed in records, discussed in interviews, and collected in observations. Understanding the "why" of the target behavior is the ultimate goal of FBA. Without a focused target behavior, it will be difficult to complete the tasks necessary to understand behavior and implement effective behavioral strategies. No doubt, this is a critical part of the *Process* phase. Before any of this elicits concern, let us reassure you. If you have reached the point in which the FBA process is necessary for a student, then the target behaviors should be straightforward and easy to identify. Perhaps the practitioner's greater challenge will be to define them.

## Strategy One: Understand the Basics

When we last saw you at Good Hope Elementary School, you were having a conversation with Donny Data, the behavior interventionist. He has now been talking for fifteen minutes about target behaviors.
"Does that make sense?" he asks. "You seem confused."
You smile and nod, "Yes, I am confused, and no, it doesn't make sense."

When we first considered training professionals in behavior planning, it seemed advantageous to start at the most basic understanding of behavior. We would like to follow that same method here. So, we will begin with the most fundamental of concepts.

© Springer International Publishing Switzerland 2016
S. M. Hadaway, A. W. Brue, *Practitioner's Guide to Functional Behavioral Assessment,*
Autism and Child Psychopathology Series, DOI 10.1007/978-3-319-23721-3_4

## *What Is a Behavior?*

A behavior is a measurable action or act. It is not a feeling. It is not an emotion. It is what a person is doing. As any language arts teacher might explain, it is a verb.

Scenario: Albert is eating an apple.

Behavior: Eating.

Scenario: Joan is kicking the ball.

Behavior: Kicking.

People are doing things all around you at all times. As practitioners, we are often asked to observe interfering behaviors. Rarely, if ever, has anyone asked us to observe a student because of his/her exemplary behavior or unbelievably good social skills. Rather, we are asked to observe the student struggling with some aspect of school appropriate behavior. When faced with challenging behaviors as a focal point, we are sometimes guilty of seeing all behaviors in those terms. If you are like us, you might momentarily forget that behavior entails actions that we sometimes describe as good or positive.

Scenario: Nelson is studying for his test.

Behavior: Studying.

Scenario: Ladonna is raising her hand.

Behavior: Raising.

This is an important distinction in a book about FBA. As a practitioner, the goal of behavior planning is not to just eliminate unwanted behavior. It is also to develop pro-social behaviors. We want to teach the individuals we support socially valid or replacement behaviors (Jolivette et al. 2000). Remember, behavior runs the full gamut, from positive to neutral to negative. It is true the behaviors that you will be focusing on will be interfering. However, be careful not to eliminate all the positive and neutral behaviors from your awareness.

Before the end of this chapter, we are going to introduce a list of words to categorize difficult behaviors. We created it for training purposes to help delineate the sometimes-subtle differences between behaviors. We hope it offers the practitioner a set of generalized groupings for clarification purposes only. Although some of these behaviors might be interfering in the classroom or at a work-training program, they are not qualitatively "bad."

Right out of college, I (Stephanie) worked as a case manager with adults who had cognitive impairments. Some of them had also been identified as having a mental illness. Within this population, our organization served a group of older individuals who had been institutionalized almost their entire lives. These individuals had only participated in a community-based training and residential program for a few years. They had decades of institutionalization and only a handful of years within the community. All of them still exhibited atypical behaviors that are more commonly seen within an institutionalized setting. These behaviors are generally unusual and might make some people uncomfortable.

One day, I took an adult male with a history of long-term institutionalization to his ophthalmologist appointment. This man was in his 60s, essentially nonverbal and imposing in size. When exposed to new people and new environments, he would begin to aggressively chant and rock back and forth. His voice was loud and his demeanor was unwelcoming. Although he sounded dangerous, he was not. He used the rocking and loud chanting as a way to cope with experiences that were agitating to him.

Certainly, in his residential placement and the day program he attended, this behavior was expected. However, in an ophthalmologist's very quiet waiting room, it was not. After about 5 min in this new surrounding, he began to loudly chant and rock. I sat with him for 10 min, unable to calm him as he scared every person in the waiting room. We were left completely on the other side of the waiting room while everyone else crammed themselves together as far away from us as possible. Finally, I gave up trying to comfort him. I knew he was not a danger to himself or anyone else, so I allowed him to chant as loudly as he wanted. I chose to sit beside him and read through a magazine. After about 10 more min, we were miraculously ushered into an examining room. I am sure the entire waiting room relaxed as we exited. Now, was this man loud? Yes. Was he dangerous? No. But his behavior was not appropriate for the waiting room.

As trained professionals, it is our hope that you will remember that certain behaviors that might be difficult in one environment can actually be commonplace and accepted in another environment. Certain behaviors that might be difficult in one environment can actually be encouraged in another. Behaviors that might be a problem in the classroom can be embraced in debate club, drama club, or on a sports team. Behaviors that might be comforting to a person can be scary to everyone else. This does not make the behaviors inherently "bad." It also does not make the person displaying them "bad." Teaching a student when to demonstrate a behavior is sometimes more important than eliminating the behavior altogether. According to Smith and Rivera (1993), "Educators must help students learn to discriminate among the behavioral options in each school situation and match that situation with the proper behavior pattern" (p. 24). Social and situational awareness are keys to navigating the social landscape. Many of the individuals we serve either have not developed these skills or choose not to use them.

Misconceptions about behavior abound. Sometimes it is difficult to see the behavior beyond the student. But it is important to differentiate. It is necessary to "identify the environmental events that reliably predict and maintain problem or 'interfering' behavior" (Gable et al. 2014). If not, behavior change cannot be addressed. Unfortunately, our experience has taught us that when a student exhibits interfering behaviors, these behaviors and sometimes the student is viewed negatively. Difficult is not the same as wrong or bad. Challenging is not the same as wrong or bad. So, maintaining professionalism and openness is critical when approaching behaviors.

## Strategy Two: Understand the Scope

### *If a Behavior Is an Action, Then What Is a Target Behavior?*

The target behavior is the action or act that is interfering with the student's success. There are many elements that can compete with an individual's ability to succeed both within the instructional and social aspects of the school environment or programmatic environment. These elements could be either *externally* or *internally* based. External factors might revolve around events, situations, or people, such as a specific adult talking sternly to the student during a classroom party. These factors might prompt or trigger the target behavior and might even need to be modified to accommodate the student. Internal factors are hidden. They are the attitudes, feelings, and emotions that the student or resident might be experiencing in regard to events, situations, or people. Internal factors might include genetic predispositions, mental illness, intelligence level, social ability, mental ability, and the ability to adapt just to name a few and might adapt and change from an endless number of elements, such as maturation, counseling, medication, and learning. Both external and internal factors are shaping elements of the target behaviors, but neither is actually the target behavior. If you remember, these can be both distant setting events and antecedents. You can think of the antecedents as fast triggers, the immediate thing happening before a behavior. You can think of distant setting events as slow triggers, the thing happening with a delayed behavioral response.

For training purposes, we created a checklist for identifying target behaviors. This checklist gives us a reference guide. It is meant to offer clarification and give those working with the same individual a unified understanding of the target behavior.

1. **Is it a behavior?** As noted previously, a behavior is an act or action that the student or resident exhibits. It can be seen; it is tangible. It is not a feeling, emotion, or attitude; it is not a mindset or disposition. It is an observable behavior.
2. **What are the qualities of the behavior?** A target behavior should be the actions of a student or resident which are viewed as interfering, disruptive, or problematic. Individuals with Disabilities Education Improvement Act of 2004 (IDEA 2004) specifically uses the word *interfering* to describe behavioral challenges. Along with that, we believe that a target behavior should be identifiable due to the pronounced difference between the target behavior and the behaviors of other individuals within the community. If the individual is a resident, this would be the therapeutic or supportive community. If the individual is a student, this would be the learning community. A target behavior will contain one or more of these qualifying identifiers. (Important note: If the student is in a residential or institutional environment or a self-contained classroom, do not compare the behavior to others being served in this population.)
   - *Is the behavior atypical?* The behavior should be considered in light of what would be the acceptable typical behavior for a student participating in a more typical learning environment. For instance, would this behavior be noticed, draw attention from others, or be considered unusual, weird, and/or disturbing in a community environment or general education setting?

- *Is the behavior inappropriate?* The behavior should be considered in light of what would be the acceptable appropriate behavior for a student participating in a more typical learning environment. For instance, would this behavior be noticed, draw attention from others, or be considered improper, offensive, and/or indecent in a community environment or general education setting?
- *Is the behavior interfering?* The behavior should be considered in light of what would be the acceptable normal behavior for a student participating in a more typical learning environment. For instance, would this behavior be noticed, draw attention from others, or be considered harassing, disruptive, and/or intrusive in a community environment or general education setting?
- *Is the behavior uncontrolled?* The behavior should be considered in light of what would be the acceptable controlled behavior for a student participating in a more typical learning environment. For instance, would this behavior be noticed, draw attention from others, or be considered disorderly, wild, and/or unrestrained in a community environment or general education setting?
- *Is the behavior dangerous?* The behavior should be considered in light of what would be the acceptable safe behavior for a student participating in a more typical learning environment. For instance, would this behavior be noticed, draw attention from others, or be considered violent, aggressive, and/or reckless in a community environment or general education setting?

So, let us say you have considered an individual you are serving, supporting, or teaching. You have gone through the necessary process of helping to determine where additional supports are needed in the existing classroom structure (Sayeski and Brown 2014). You were then able to identify a target behavior from the criteria listed above. The only problem is that the individual you are serving, supporting, or teaching does not just exhibit one behavior that meets the criteria, but four or five behaviors. What then? Do you complete an FBA on every behavior that meets these criteria?

In theory, you might be able to answer yes to this question. In all practicality, however, this would be a time-consuming process that would eventually make any intervention weaker or even ineffective. In order to effectively address behavioral concerns, it is important to become more selective in identifying target behaviors. As a general rule, one to three behaviors should be selected. For more information, see our Target Behavior Help Sheet in Appendix C.

> Let's take a break and return to Good Hope Elementary School. You spent forty-five minutes with Donny Data, and you have identified six behaviors that Willow Wilding really, really needs to resolve. You are working on these behaviors when you come across your notes on Donny's criteria. He told you to pick one to three behaviors. You stare hopelessly at your notes. Which behaviors do you select?

Selection does not have to be a difficult task. Sometimes, it is just as simple as organizing your data and asking a few questions. In order to help you with this process, we have used our behaviors from above to act as prompt questions for guidance. These might be beneficial when working collaboratively to keep the discussion focused on the more prominent and extreme behaviors. Prior to looking at those, there are three additional qualifiers to consider: intensity, frequency, and duration.

## Which Behaviors Have the Greatest Degree of Intensity?

When considering the intensity of a behavior, the practitioner is determining the level of severity in which the behavior is demonstrated. For the purposes of the target behavior, we will define intensity on two different scales. The first is on a continuum ranging from mild to moderate to severe.

*Mild* The behavior demonstrated is interfering, challenging, atypical, and/or disruptive, such as drumming on a desk or humming loudly. The behavior is not aggressive or dangerous.

*Moderate* The behavior demonstrated is verbally threatening; destructive to objects and/or items; and/or mildly, physically aggressive such as a small push or shove. The behavior might entail pushing over a desk or tearing up an assignment.

*Severe* The behavior demonstrated is physically aggressive to the extent of intending or actually causing harm to others. The behavior might entail punching a student in the face or throwing a desk at the teacher.

The second scale rates the intensity from 1 to 5. It also focuses on the scope of the behavior, but takes into account other people present.

1—The behavior interferes with only the student or resident.
2—The behavior interferes with other individuals in the immediate area surrounding the student or resident.
3—The behavior interferes with all individuals in the room with the student or resident.
4—The behavior interferes with individuals both inside the room and in the immediate areas outside of the room, such as the hallway, other rooms, or other therapeutic groups.
5—The behavior interferes with individuals throughout the building. The behavior contains an element of danger or impending harm to others.

Either scale is acceptable for consideration. The team determining the target behaviors can use one or both. The team can also create their own. Priority should be given to the most severe behaviors.

## Which Behaviors Are Most Frequent?

When considering the frequency of a behavior, the practitioner is determining how often the behavior occurs. The target behavior should occur with a degree of frequency. Although the amount of frequency might be somewhat dependent on the context of the behavior, it is assumed that a behavior that has only occurred once or twice is not a chronic problem. When considering identifying target behaviors, we recommend focusing on behaviors that occur weekly. (Severe behaviors or those that cause harm are definitely exceptions to this understanding.)

## Which Behaviors Have the Longest Span of Duration?

When considering the duration of a behavior, the practitioner is determining how long the behavior occurs. Even small behaviors, such as tapping a pencil on a desk, can become significantly interfering if they occur continually over a span of time. When considering identifying target behaviors, our general rule of thumb is to consider any behavior that occurs for 15 min or more without stopping.

Part of determining which behaviors should be target behaviors is achieving a balance between intensity, frequency, and duration. For instance, we have suggested a good measuring point for frequency in the behaviors that occur weekly. We qualify that here. If a behavior occurs monthly and is harmful to others, this severity outweighs the previous measuring point. Although we cannot account for every level of severity, duration, and frequency, we can advocate that when a severe behavior is reoccurring and unresolved, it should go to the proverbial "top of the list." Physical danger and harm to others takes precedence over less aggressive behaviors.

However, there are times when a student or resident has one incident of significantly at-risk behavior. The student or resident might have gotten into a fight. Even though this behavior might have been severe enough to warrant extreme consequences, carefully consider if this should be a target behavior. Certainly, preventive measures should be taken. In fact, the team might want to put a safety plan into place. If the safety plan and other preventive measures work and the behavior does not reappear, then it should not be a target behavior. The consequences enacted might be all that the individual needs to resolve the behavior of concern.

### *Clarifying Questions*

Below we have listed a few more questions to help you refine your list of possible target behaviors. You only need one to three target behaviors. When using this list, think of a typical community or classroom setting. What would the target behavior look like in a more typical environment? If you have more than three behaviors you are considering, ask:

- *Which behaviors are the most atypical?*
- *Which behaviors are the most inappropriate?*
- *Which behaviors are the most interfering?*
- *Which behaviors are the most uncontrolled?*
- *Which behaviors are the most dangerous?*

Remember to use *no more than three* of the most intense, frequent, and ongoing behaviors. The practitioner's or team's goal should be to strike a balance between frequency, duration, and intensity. As you work through the selection process, be careful to discriminate between these three. If only one behavior is significant enough to need FBA, then use only one behavior.

## Strategy Three: What to Do

At this point, one to three target behaviors have been identified. So, to effectively address the behavior, the target behavior needs to be defined. Identifying and operationalizing a target behavior is essential to the accuracy of both the FBA and the behavioral intervention plans (BIP; Conroy et al. 2009). To develop an effective target behavior, it must first be operationalized. When you operationalize a behavior, you are defining it in observable and measurable terms. Anyone who reads the target behavior will understand the parameters within which the behavior presents. There is a general consensus about certain aspects of an operationalized definition. Most would agree that an operationalized, target behavior will:

- Be specific
- Be descriptive
- Have an observable beginning and end
- Have a measurable dimension

Additionally, one could add:

- Understandable
- Relevant to the context
- Objective

## Strategy Four: Application

So, how do you actually write a target behavior? Keeping in mind the practices above, ask yourself these simple questions:

1. *Who?*
2. *What?*
3. *When?*

And sometimes…

4. *How?*

That might seem less than concrete, so we are going to give you some examples of what we mean.

### *Refusals*

Let us take a look at a student. Mark refuses to work in Math class. When he is given an assignment, he does not pick up his pencil to begin. If he is told to begin by his teacher, Mark often tells the teacher "No."

Too vague: Mark (who) *refuses* to do his work (what).

Ask: How does he refuse? What does his refusals look like? When do his refusals occur?

Target behavior: Mark (who) refuses and verbally states "No" (what) when prompted to complete math computation problems (when).

## Physical Aggressive Behavior

Ava is physically aggressive. She does not handle frustration or disappointment well. When she does poorly in a class or even loses at a game, she will often lash out at other students by kicking or hitting them.

Too vague: Ava is aggressive towards her classmates.

Ask: How is she aggressive? What does her aggression look like? With whom is she aggressive? When does this aggression occur?

Target behavior: Ava hits and kicks other students when she experiences a disappointment, setback, or loss.

## Out-of-Area Behavior

Juan appears very restless. He will remain in his seat during individual assignments. However, when placed in a group, he often leaves his seat. He will wander around the room, sometimes running and skipping.

Too vague: Juan wanders around the room.

Ask: What does the wandering behavior look like? When does this behavior occur? What is the actual problem? Is it that he moves around the room? There are times when moving around the room is permissible. So, is it that he is wandering around without permission?

Target behavior: Juan leaves his assigned area in groups without permission.

## Disruptive Behavior

Carla does not like to read. Every time her class begins to read, Carla starts talking out to the teacher. She will talk about unrelated topics, such as going to the movies. She will also talk on topic about the reading assignment. Even when she talks on topic, Carla delays reading instruction. When her teacher attempts to move on, Carla will become louder and more demanding.

Too vague: Carla is disruptive in reading.

Ask: How is she disruptive? What does her disruptive behavior look like? With whom is she disruptive? When does this disruption occur?

Target behavior: Carla talks out both on and off topic to her teacher throughout her reading lessons.

To write a clear, target behavior, ask clarifying questions:

- Is this specific?
- Is this descriptive?
- Does this behavior have an observable beginning and end?
- Does this behavior have a measurable dimension?

Additionally, one could add:

- Is this understandable?
- Is this relevant to the context?
- Is this objective?

## Strategy Five: What Not to Do

**Avoid Vague Descriptions** One pitfall in developing a successful target behavior is to be vague. It is easy to use broad terms. But, remember, it is important for the behavior to be specific and measurable.

Here are some common terms that are too broad and vague:

- Aggressive
- Disruptive
- Tantrums
- Outbursts
- Inattentive
- Off-task
- All emotion/feeling words: depressed, sad, angry, disappointed, mad, upset, and frustrated
- Avoids
- Psychotic
- Hyperactive
- Destructive

The difficulty with these terms is that they are neither descriptive nor measurable. How do you measure a feeling? For example:

- A student becomes angry. Well, what does the anger look like? For this student, anger might be screaming out profanity or throwing items in the room. Anger cannot be measured, but screaming out profanity and throwing items in a classroom can be.
- A student becomes destructive. What does the destruction look like? Destruction cannot be measured, but breaking objects or tearing up objects can be measured.
- A student becomes depressed. What does depression look like? Is the student crying or laying her head on her desk? These behaviors can be measured.

**Avoid Writing Goals** It is important to remember that the target behavior is not a goal. In both treatment and academic planning, practitioners set goals for residents and students. These are examples of goals:

*Goal Scenario 1:* During whole-group instruction, Evan will refrain from talking out with two or less prompts.

*Goal Scenario 2:* During transitions, Ellen will remain with her group 100% of the time.

A goal is the desired behavior that you want to see; it is the optimal situation. For example, *Evan will no longer talk in whole-group instruction* or *Ellen will remain with her group during transitions.* Conversely, a target behavior is the problematic action or act that the student is exhibiting.

*Target Behavior Scenario 1:* Evan talks out off topic during whole-group instruction.

*Target Behavior Scenario 2:* Ellen leaves her assigned area without permission during transition times.

> It is the day of Willow Wilding's meeting. The team has had a good review of Willow's records and data. After some debate, her target behaviors have been written.
> First try: Target Behavior One: Willow is destructive. (Too vague. What does she destroy? How does she destroy it?)
> Second try: Target Behavior One: Destructive behavior—Willow uses her hands and feet to turn over furniture, such as desks and chairs, tear items off the wall, and rip up items, such as schoolwork, books and papers throughout her school day.
> First try: Target Behavior Two: Out of Area Behavior—Willow runs around the room and we can't get her to sit down.
> Second try: Target Behavior Two: Out of Area Behavior—Willow leaves her assigned area without permission throughout her school day.
> You smile. This might just work.

# A Before-You-Proceed Checklist

1. Understand what a behavior is.
2. Identify the selection process for target behaviors.
3. Understand intensity, frequency, and duration.
4. Understand that a target behavior must be operationalized and what that means.
5. Understand how to apply who, what, when, and how to the development of target behaviors.
6. Know how to avoid vague descriptions for target behaviors.

**Author Takeaways**

*Takeaway from Stephanie, the behavior specialist:*

The target behavior is the beginning of the FBA. The success of strategies and interventions used with the student is dependent on the accuracy of that description. Most errors that I have seen involve being too vague. A good target behavior will be understandable to anyone who reads it. They will know what the behavior actually looks like. By giving a clear and measurable definition, you have taken the first step towards a successful FBA.

*Takeaway from Alan, the school psychologist:*

Specificity is my main point from this chapter. As a school psychologist who completes many psychoeducational evaluations each year, I receive and review many referrals. The referring problem sometimes is too vague. When I ask a teacher to be more specific, the information I receive is more "rich" and helpful. The same applies to the FBA process; I need to know specifics before I am able to offer any feedback that is likely to assist in changing a student's behavior.

# References

Conroy, M. A., Alter, P. J., & Scott, T. M. (2009). Functional behavioral assessment and students with emotional/behavioral disorder: When research, policy, and practice collide. In T. E. Scruggs & M. A. Mastropieri (Eds.), *Policy and practice: Advances in learning and behavioral disabilities* (pp. 133–167). Bradford: Emerald Group Publishing.

Gable, R. A., Park, K. L., & Scott, T. M. (2014). Functional behavioral assessment and students at risk for or with emotional disabilities: Current issues and considerations. *Education and Treatment of Children, 37*(1), 111–135.

Jolivette, K., Scott, T. M., & Nelson, C. M. (2000). The link between functional behavior assessments (FBAs) and behavioral intervention plans (BIPs). *ERIC Digest, E592*, EDO-00-1.

Losinski, M., Maag, J. W., Katsiyannis, A., & Ryan, J. B. (2015). The use of structural behavioral assessment to develop interventions for secondary students exhibiting challenging behaviors. *Education and Treatment of Children, 38*(2), 149–174.

Sayeski, K. L., & Brown, M. R. (2014). Developing a classroom management plan using a tiered approach. *Teaching Exceptional Children, 47*(2), 119–127.

Smith, D. D., & Rivera, D. M. (1993). *Effective discipline* (2nd ed.). Austin: Pro-Ed.

# Chapter 5
# Process: Record Review

## What You Need to Know

For just a moment, let us revisit the phase we are in. At this point, you have prepared for the functional behavioral assessment (FBA) and have a preliminary definition for target behaviors. We stipulate preliminary definition(s) because information that is gained through both indirect and direct methods of data collection might mandate that we change, modify, or even add definitions for the target behavior. Next, the practitioner begins data collection. In the Process phase, if the target behavior is the definition of what you are searching for, then data collection is the product of that search.

Data collection is a term that is used frequently in educational, behavioral, and research circles. For some beginners, visions of white coats, clipboards, and sterile laboratories might guide their notions and stir their concerns. For others, the idea of data collection might conjure images of drinking lots and lots of coffee to avoid sleep while searching through countless journals and reference books. For even others, those two words can strike fear by reminding them that data collection can be used to evaluate performance.

Knowledge acquisition has been noted to be an important starting point in the professional development of school personnel (Bergstrom 2008; Crone et al. 2007; Kratochwill et al. 2007). When training teachers and practitioners, we have found that many of them cringe at the mere mention of the words *data collection*. Mostly, they seem to dread data collection because they are not exactly sure what to do when it comes to behavioral data collecting. They can quickly tell you how to gather data on reading progress or math attainment, but behavior seems to illicit a sort of dreaded pause. Understanding this, our goal is to make this as easy to understand as possible.

© Springer International Publishing Switzerland 2016
S. M. Hadaway, A. W. Brue, *Practitioner's Guide to Functional Behavioral Assessment,*
Autism and Child Psychopathology Series, DOI 10.1007/978-3-319-23721-3_5

## Strategy One: Understand the Basics

> It is the day after Willow Wilding's meeting. You have two target behaviors that are opera-
> tionalized. Willow's parents were pleased. Mrs. Huffing actually smiled at you today and
> you believe that you might have this under control.
> After school, you are looking through your notes. During your meeting with Donny Data,
> he told you to begin collecting data once the target behavior had been operationalized. You
> think you can do that with no problem. You collect data all the time. But wait! Is behavioral
> data gathering different than what you've done in the past? Goodness, how do you collect
> data on behavior?

Data collection is basically gathering information. In the case of FBA, the information gathered is on the identified target behavior(s).

Within the context of FBA, there are two means to collect data that we will
discuss. First, there is *indirect observational data*. This information comes from
secondary sources, such as parents, teachers, administrators, and caregivers. It is the
information that is gleaned from interviews, records, and informal assessments. The
challenge for the practitioner is information from interviews, and informal assessments is subjective; therefore, the reliability and validity are questionable (Martella
et al. 2012). Second, there is *direct observational data*. This is the information you
gather. It is the first-hand recordings of the student's behavior derived from observation. It does not come from secondary sources; it comes from data that you have
collected. Using both indirect and direct forms of data collection aids the practitioner in objectivity and understanding.

Let us review quickly: Indirect methods of data collecting are from secondary
sources, whereas direct methods of data collecting are from first-hand observations.
Over the next several chapters, we are going to take you through each of these methods. For now, we will start with reviewing records.

## Strategy Two: Understand the Scope

We promised to make this as simple as possible. So, let us answer an obvious question.

## *What Are Records?*

A record is a type of documentation that contains information regarding one or
many aspects of a person.

## *Since We Are Focusing on Behavior, Do We Only Review Disciplinary Records?*

No, typically disciplinary records will focus on the actions that occurred when the student or resident broke a rule. Disciplinary records offer important information, but the practitioner has the responsibility of viewing the individual through a wider scope than just the individual's infractions and the administrative responses to those infractions. A disciplinary record is part of a records review. It is just not the only part.

## *So, What Else Should Be Reviewed?*

In order to gain both a current and historical perspective of the student, the practitioner should approach records reviews thoroughly. This type of review should be systematic (Barnhill 2005). We have compiled the types of records that might be available on a student or resident. Depending on age, condition, and the institution in which they are being served, every student or resident might not have records in all of these areas.

*Attendance Records* An attendance record contains the documentation of how many days a person has attended the institution in question. Treatment centers, schools, work sites, day programs, and residential programs will all have some form of attendance documentation. Additionally, there might be attendance records that encompass participation. If the individual has been asked to attend a social skills class or a therapeutic group, their attendance in these programmatic opportunities should also be gathered.

*Medical History* A medical record contains the medical history of the student or resident. Medical records would consist of medical diagnoses, medications, treatment, and other physical conditions. Even if a condition has been resolved, it is important to note surgeries or other treatments that occurred with a medical condition. If the school or program the individual is attending has a clinic or nurse, it would be advantageous to check and see how often the individual had visited the clinic or nurse.

*Disciplinary Records* A disciplinary record often contains administrative or office referrals for infractions, results of the office or administrative visit, number of days suspended from the school or program, information on referrals to tribunals or disciplinary boards, police reports, and expulsion information.

*Academic History* An academic record review would involve reviewing the student's grades, achievement, and other notable academic information. As the student ages, this history will be more diverse. Take into account times when the student has had successes, such as honor roll. If the student's performance has changed during his/her educational career, this information should be highlighted. If the individual is in a residential or treatment facility, academic history remains important. For teenagers and adults, be sure to determine the last level of education that was completed. If an individual's academic career prematurely ended, investigate the reasons why this happened.

*Assessment Records* An assessment record entails a wide range of testing data. Standardized state testing, placement testing, or diagnostic testing can all be considered when conducting an assessment review. Although typical weekly and classroom testing is unnecessary, be certain to attain the student's current level of academic functioning when reviewing academic records and interviewing teachers. If the student has become eligible for additional services, such as special education, this testing could also be considered.

*Individualized Education Program (IEP)* If an individual attending the public education system has been identified as having a disability, he or she has an IEP. A review of the IEP would entail the following: goals, interventions, the behavior intervention plan, extended school year services, accommodations, modifications, testing information, service hours, and programs for student supports, such as speech language, occupational therapy, or physical therapy. The IEP also gives valuable insight into past testing and the student's current level of functioning.

## Strategy Three: What to Do

Prior to beginning a thorough review of the student or resident's records, you need to ascertain your level of access to these documents. An individual's educational and treatment information is protected by both privacy and confidentiality. If the student has an IEP, the information contained in this legal document is not public domain. Only certain individuals have a right to review the document. If you are not the student's teacher or case manager, be certain to understand your access limitations. But not just the IEP, it is necessary for you to treat all student records in this manner. Additionally, any resident involved in a therapeutic program also has rights to privacy and confidentiality. Before proceeding with a review, gain the necessary consent to examine all documents. Remember, just because you work in a school or treatment center does not guarantee you access to these documents. For both ethical and legal reasons, follow protocol for your organization, and if in doubt, gain consent. It is better to do so unnecessarily than to go forward and find out that you were not authorized to view certain information. For more information, check out this side-by-side presentation of Individuals with Disabilities Education Act (IDEA) and Family Educational Rights and Privacy Act (FERPA) at https://www2. ed.gov/policy/gen/guid/ptac/pdf/idea-ferpa.pdf.

Beyond your place of employment, you might need additional information to review records. When you need to gain access to records, such as medical history, you will need to gain consent from the parent/guardian or consent from the individual if he/she is an adult. In these instances, you will need to secure a release of information. A release of information allows the doctor, hospital, therapist, or treatment center (to name just a few) to send you requested information regarding the individual. The individual (adult) or parent/guardian (minor) signs the release of information. Without this signature, the information cannot be released to you. As part of the release, there needs to be a clear statement of informational parameters. This will define the information you are seeking. Physicians and other mental health professionals have a responsibility to legally give you only the information that is requested. So, be aware of the information that you are requesting on the release form.

Although there are many aspects of reviewing a student's records that might seem obvious, we still felt that it might be beneficial to offer a few suggestions that have served us well over the years.

First, look for standouts. When reading through these documents, take note of exceptions. Consistent school attendance is probably common for most students. When a student is excessively absent, that should stand out. Does the student or resident take medication? If so, for what reason and for how long? Does the student or resident have some type of medical condition or genetic condition? You want to make note of any condition, situation, or behavior that is atypical or uncommon.

Second, look for changes. Life events, grades that drop, an outgoing student who suddenly becomes extremely shy, these are all significant changes. When reviewing data, do not miss the times that the student or resident experienced or exhibited a change. Changes that occur to the person can impact behavior. Changes that occur because of the person can indicate an underlying issue that might need further investigation.

Third, look for patterns. By identifying patterns in behavior, the practitioner can begin to understand the underlying context of behaviors and give the team an investigative area within the occurrences of challenging behaviors (Moreno and Bullock 2011). Within a thorough records review, you would want to look for repetition in behavior, times, seasons, and environment. Every January, does the resident go to the nurse frequently? During math class, is the student receiving a disciplinary referral? If you notice a pattern but do not understand it, that is okay. A student might be disrupting the math class because he has a skill deficit and cannot do the work. Or a student could be disrupting the math class because he does not like the teacher or the student who sits next to him. When this occurs, simply use the interview process to clarify the pattern you have detected in documentation. This is an excellent way to link multiple sources of information for greater understanding.

Fourth, look for strategies, goals, and interventions that have been tried. There might be strategies that have worked; there might be strategies that have not worked. As you move through the paperwork, try to identify any progress or lack of progress in this arena. This is a vital aspect of behavior planning and will also serve to make you well informed.

## Strategy Four: Application

There are many documents that you will want to examine as part of this process. If you are working with a specific timeline, it is important to use your time wisely. As with every method we advocate, this is what has worked for us. If your organization or system mandates different methods, please use those. We have found that reviewing records is often done hastily or sometimes not at all. The vast amount of information available causes some practitioners to delay a records review. We encourage you to begin this process prior to an FBA. When you have your first meeting, you should have already reviewed the documents available to you in your building. Certainly, gaining consent and a release of information will be needed in some instances as well as for information that has to be obtained from other sources. The first meeting is a great place to do those follow-up events, but do not put off examining what is legally available to you as soon as possible. This will help to make the process easier.

We have created a few steps that have always helped us organize this process:

1. Determine your legal and procedural right to access the individual's records in your building or organization.
2. Follow any procedural requirements to obtain these records.
3. Review the individual's records in your building or from your organization in which you have legal and procedural rights to access.
4. Meet with the parent or adult individual (this could also take place in your first meeting with the team).
5. Gain consent and release of information to access records from outside sources that are pertinent to the FBA.
6. Gain and obtain access to records from outside sources that are pertinent to the FBA.
7. Review records in an area where no one who does not hold legal or procedural rights to view the information is present.
8. Note any standouts, changes, patterns, strategies, interventions, goals, or programming that is relevant to the FBA process.
9. Follow up with questions regarding the records in the interview process.
10. Successfully link sources of information to gain greater understanding of the individual's behavior.

> You have just finished Willow Wilding's records review. "That went well!" you think to yourself. You had printed off a list you made so you wouldn't forget anything.
> Attendance
> Medical
> Disciplinary
> IEP
> Yep, you completed everything. And Willow Wilding's records were somewhat easy to go through. You look over your notes. Willow has perfect attendance, so the consistency is good. She doesn't have any outstanding medical issues. It is clear, though, that she has numerous office referrals. And it is interesting that the majority of those referrals occurred in the afternoon; there were very few that took place in the morning. Even though her

records indicate that she moves and leaves the room without permission, at least 95 % of her disciplinary referrals were for destructive behaviors, such as tearing items apart. You make a note to keep this in mind.

Tomorrow, Gwen Gillespie will begin her part of this team FBA. You think aloud for just a moment, "She agreed to do the interviews and the observations when I momentarily panicked yesterday. She is really a great lead special education teacher! I wonder if there is a reason she is not responding to my emails...."

## A Before-You-Proceed Checklist

1. Understand the meaning of data collection.
2. Understand what constitutes an indirect method of data collecting.
3. Know the importance of confidentiality, privilege, consent, and release of information.
4. Identify the different types of records that might be available on a student or a resident.
5. Identify four areas to review when examining records.

**Author Takeaways**
*Takeaway from Stephanie, the behavioral specialist:*
Reviewing a student or a resident's records can be overwhelming. Often, there are multiples of everything that have accumulated over the years. There are multiple goals, strategies, disciplinary reports, assessments, and academic information. It might be challenging to wade through all the historical details that are part of an individual's record. Even though it is challenging, make it a priority. If a student has transferred many times in their school career, a significant amount of valuable information could have been overlooked. I have personally found information that was critical in effective behavior planning buried in documentation that was overlooked or ignored in a new school setting. Patterns of absence or illness often indicate deficits that need to be addressed for the student to succeed behaviorally. If a practitioner does not examine the records thoroughly, it can leave gaps in understanding that might prevent the progress everyone hopes for with a struggling student. Make the time to do a thorough review of the records!
*Takeaway from Alan, the school psychologist:*
As a school psychologist, I find it imperative to review all available records. I need to understand the child holistically if I am able to provide assistance. Records may include many keys to helping the child; experience will help you to not only know what to look for but also to recognize a piece of information that may otherwise have been overlooked. Granted, a cursory review of records is better than no review at all, but it is important to set aside time in which to go over all of the information you have available to you.

# References

Barnhill, G. P. (2005). Functional behavioral assessment in schools. *Intervention in School and Clinic, 40*(3), 131–143.

Bergstrom, M. K. (2008). Professional development in response to intervention: Implementation of a model in a rural region. *Rural Special Education Quarterly, 27*(4), 27–36.

Crone, D. A., Hawken, L. S., & Bergstrom, M. K. (2007). A demonstration of training, implementing, and using functional behavioral assessment in 10 elementary and middle school settings. *Journal of Positive Behavior Interventions, 9*(1), 15–29.

Kratochwill, T. R., Volpiansky, P., Clements, M., & Ball, C. (2007). Professional development in implementing and sustaining multitier prevention models: Implications for response to intervention. *School Psychology Review, 36*(4), 618–631.

Martella, R. C., Nelson, J. R., Marchand-Martella, N. E., & O'Reilly, M. (2012). *Comprehensive behavior management: Individualized, classroom, and schoolwide*. Thousand Oaks: Sage Publications.

Moreno, G., & Bullock, L. M. (2011). Principles of positive behaviour supports: Using the FBA as a problem-solving approach to address challenging behaviours beyond special populations. *Emotional and Behavioural Difficulties, 16*(2), 117–127.

# Chapter 6
# Process: Interviews

## What You Need to Know

In our last chapter, we identified two types of data collection, direct observational data collection and indirect observational data collection. Just as reviewing records is a type of indirect method of gaining information, so is the interviewing process. As you might remember, collecting data in an indirect method means that the information you gather comes from secondary sources, such as parents, teachers, administrators, and caregivers.

Prior to proceeding with this chapter, we feel it is important to add a few cautionary words. Information gained from interviews, as has been noted, is subjective. Floyd et al. (2005) report that interviews are limited to the recollections of informants and their personal judgments. In this regard, the practitioner must guard against misleading information. Certainly, information gathered in interviews, questionnaires, surveys, checklists, and any other type of informal assessment provides unique insights into the individual. The practitioner should remember not to rely on the interviews alone; direct observational data are needed (Martella et al. 2012).

## Strategy One: Understand the Basics

Gwen Gillespie had met Mr. and Mrs. Wilding at the door and escorted them to her office. She had set out some mints and chocolate candy. Mr. and Mrs. Wilding each took a water bottle and the three talked a few minutes about the weather.

After about five minutes, Gwen leaned forward and smiled, "I am so glad the two of you could make it today. All of this takes time, but it is all for Willow. There might be some tough questions here, but take your time. Before we get started, do you have any questions for me?"

Drew Wilding nodded. "We understand this is confidential, but what does that really mean in a school? We don't have anything to hide, but we are private."

Gwen nodded. "I understand. Let me explain it to you."

© Springer International Publishing Switzerland 2016

S. M. Hadaway, A. W. Brue, *Practitioner's Guide to Functional Behavioral Assessment,*
Autism and Child Psychopathology Series, DOI 10.1007/978-3-319-23721-3_6

In Chap. 1, we discussed the implications for maintaining appropriate, professional conduct. We would like to begin our discussion with these implications.

Professionally, we have learned that a successful interview begins long before the practitioner asks a parent, teacher, or student the first question on a form. It begins the first moment the practitioner has contact with a parent, teacher, or student. Within a practitioner's workday, there are many opportunities to build relationships with parents, coworkers, and the referring institutions. These relationships are often key to building rapport and trust. Rapport and trust help to lower barriers that others might exhibit when sharing information. Parents might be protective of a child's medical information and demonstrate reluctance to share it. Teachers might be concerned that admitting some of their management struggles with a student reflects poorly on their abilities. Administrators might be worried that explaining the extent of the student's problem behavior might prompt you to demand strategies or interventions that stretch their overworked personnel. Without establishing professional rapport and professional trust, critical information might remain undisclosed.

For the practitioner, interactions with others shape their willingness to disclose personal and sometimes unflattering information to you. Meetings, direct observations, and records reviews can all be impacted by these interactive experiences. However, the interview is the part of functional behavioral assessment (FBA) that is probably most impacted by relational experiences.

In the interview, the practitioner and interviewee are entering into a series of exchanges that will add to the storehouse of data collected on a student's behavior. Therefore, it is important to prepare for the fullest possible exchange. In our opinion, professionalism is the cornerstone for building a successful, informational exchange.

*Professionalism Involves Conduct* Dress code, language, and behavior are areas in which people might judge professionals. Sometimes, outside contractors or professionals who are not employed within an institution or organization are more mindful of environmental expectations than those who work daily within the institution or organization. Thus, they tend to exhibit more restraint when in this new environment. If you are or you are not an employee of the school, treatment program or organization in which you are conducting an FBA, your behavior should exemplify professional conduct. If the level of professionalism of others lessens in more familiar environments, guard against this. When you enter the premises, it is important to conduct yourself in accordance with the policies that govern the environment. Whether in dress code, language, or behavior, your conduct should match or exceed a standard of behavior that the institution you are working in would uphold.

*Professionalism Involves Readiness* If an interviewer is tardy, absent, or comes to the interview unprepared, it can significantly impact the information gained from the interview. Your level of readiness indicates to the person you are interviewing that you care about the information that you are asking of them. It is much easier to give information to someone who cares than to someone who is careless.

*Professionalism Involves Objectivity* It is important to be aware of cultural values and differences. When interviewing others, your own biases, values, and preferences should not enter into the interview setting. Refrain from value-laden questions and commentary. You are not interviewing to correct, teach, or change. You are interviewing to hear, learn, and gain data regarding the behavior, preferences, and needs of the student or resident exhibiting behavior. Any extraneous information that contains your own bias or does not impact the behavior of the student in some manner should be left alone.

*Professionalism Involves Confidentiality* The data that you gain should be treated as confidential. The information that the interviewee shares with you should not be accessible to everyone in the environment. It should only be used in the development of the FBA and the behavior intervention plan (BIP). When you have gained non-pertinent information from any secondary source, do not include it in your reporting. Everything shared in the interview will not be necessary for the FBA or behavior planning. Be selective and mindful of private matters, and do not unnecessarily include them. In the event that the student/resident or family member discloses information regarding abuse, suicidal intent, or homicidal intent, then you should act in the best interests of the student/resident. It is important to understand your legal responsibilities regarding reporting abuse or threatening statements prior to the interview. Policies, law, and ethical standards govern this area. Do not enter an interview without understanding your legal and ethical responsibilities regarding abuse, suicidal threats, or homicidal threats. If you ever encounter this type of serious situation, you will want to feel confident in knowing the correct protocol to follow.

## Strategy Two: Understand the Scope

As you can probably tell by now, we believe that there is far more to the interviewing process than just picking up a quick questionnaire and asking a few questions. An effective interview can help you determine a functional relationship between the target behavior and maintaining contingencies (Cipani and Schock 2010). An effective interview can also help in your operational definition of the target behavior. The interview is always a good time to revisit the target behavior and make sure you are on track. We actually conduct the teacher interview before finalizing the target behaviors for this very reason.

No doubt in order to obtain your current job or gain entry into an academic program, you had to go through an interview process. For just a moment, take the time to reflect on those experiences. What was the interview dynamic? What types of questions were important to the interviewer? How did you feel in this process? We believe that remembering your own experiences as an interviewee will help you to become a better interviewer. Just in case you have blocked out the experience, it seems to us that there are three elements that will help you gain the information you need.

*Setting the Atmosphere*—We are approaching the interviewing process under a major assumption: When people feel comfortable, they are more likely to remain accessible throughout the interview. Often, family members or caregivers are being asked for an interview because of disruptive or difficult behavior that the student or resident is exhibiting. Family members sometimes feel uncomfortable or, worse, accused of contributing or causing this behavior. Other times, a family member might feel protective and the need to rationalize or even justify a student or resident's behavior. If a caregiver feels guarded, defensive, or tense, their openness to the questions posed might be limited. Ultimately, this prohibits the interviewer from gaining data that might help the student or resident. Setting a comfortable and open atmosphere will help as you interview individuals associated with the FBA, including teachers, counselors, parents, and even students. We are going to offer you more concrete tips on setting the atmosphere in the next section.

*Interviewing the Right People*—It is amazing how many people can come into contact with a student throughout a school day. Each and every person might have a different experience and something to add to the FBA process. But each and every experience might not be appropriate to consider. Therefore, it is important to carefully select the individuals who need to be interviewed in regard to the student. When determining this, consider how often a person is with a student. For instance, the physical education teacher might see the student only once a week, while a science teacher might see the student every day. If the student is older and changes classes, it might be advantageous to interview all of the academic teachers as a group. If an individual, such as the counselor, a paraprofessional, or the principal, is frequently involved with the student, it might be wise to consider interviewing them as well. Always interview the parent or caregiver. The differences between home and school can further illuminate environmental factors that precipitate behavior. One word of caution: You can interview too many people. So, select people who will truly offer insight or can speak about experiences that relate to the FBA.

Above all, do not neglect to interview the student or resident. It is important that the student or resident has input into his or her own behavior, preferences, and level of functioning. When interviewed, research has indicated that students are able to provide useful and reliable information on their own behavior (Kinch et al. 2001).

As is the case with any interview, it is important to make the questions accessible to everyone. If you are interviewing an individual who is nonverbal, identified with a language disorder, identified as having symptoms related to autism, is hearing impaired, or English is not their primary language, be sure to take this all into account. Make certain to provide for these situations by having an interpreter, therapist, or teacher available for the interview. If the student is on a lower cognitive level or very young, be sure to modify the questions to make them as understandable as possible. Use pictures or other resources that will aid in the interviewing process.

In the event that you interview an individual who refuses to respond to your questions, consider alternate possibilities. You might be able to have the counselor or the teacher interview the student. Or you might want to have a familiar person give the individual a personal preference inventory.

As is the case with everyone you interview, be sure to treat the student/resident with the utmost courtesy and respect. Also, treat his or her information with the same amount of confidentiality that you would apply to anyone else. Keep in mind that you are presenting questions about the student's behavior that might not be easy to talk about. If this is a highly aggressive student, the questions might trigger an aggressive response. Use good judgment when determining the types of questions that will be asked.

On a final, cautionary note: *It is best to interview the student or resident after the observations are nearing completion.* Interviewing the student prior to observing them could greatly impact your direct observational data results.

*Asking the Right Questions*—We begin this section with another major assumption: Every question is not a good question. There are some types of information that are personal, interesting, and completely irrelevant to the process. Stay away from these types of questions. Focus on the information that is needed. Avoid the prying, frivolous, and unnecessary data collecting. Find the questions that are relevant to the situation at hand and ask those questions. Floyd et al. (2005) state:

> Although the information derived from interviews is comprised of third parties and is one person's perspective, when collected through the use of objectively phrased questioning, it can still provide critical information on the possible operation of the behavior and can be used to identify possible replacement behavior for the eventual BIP. (p. 121)

To assist you in the interview process, we have included a Parent/Caregiver Questionnaire in Appendix D, a Staff/Personnel Questionnaire in Appendix E, and a Student Questionnaire in Appendix F. They are thorough and were designed to ask a range of questions applicable to the purposes of both the FBA and BIP. Many questions are brief, so do not be concerned about the length. There might be questions that are not applicable to your current situation. Therefore, it is a good idea to review the form prior to asking the questions. Depending on the information you are gathering, the interview on average should take between 30 min and an hour. Be sure to check them out.

## Strategy Three: What to Do

Structure is key when following an interview format. Umbreit et al. (2006) list a series of structured questions that focus on the behaviors of concern. By keeping the interview focused with structured questions, the practitioner is more likely to obtain reliable information. Additionally, there are certain elements that are important to address regarding behavior. Most interviews can be divided into five categories: behaviors, setting events, antecedents, consequences, and interventions (O'Neill et al. 1996).

In order to address these principles, we are going to cover eight areas of focus that will allow the practitioner to obtain behavioral data from the interviewee. These areas are topography, characteristics, pervasiveness, history/conditions, environmental conditions, interventions, function, and preferences.

*Topography* It is important to identify what the target behaviors look like to the person you are interviewing. This is called the topography.

*Characteristics* Additionally, identify the impression the person you are interviewing has of the characteristics of the target behavior. Do these behaviors seem atypical, inappropriate, interfering, uncontrolled, and/or dangerous?

*Pervasiveness* Along with these, it is important to understand the frequency, intensity, and duration of the behavior. How frequently does the behavior occur? This can range from multiple times in an hour to monthly. How intense is the behavior? This can range from mildly disruptive to causing physical injury to someone. Finally, what is the duration of the behavior? This can range from a few seconds to ongoing throughout the day.

*History/Conditions* The interview is an excellent time to clarify any information from the individual's records. Also, it is important to use the interview to learn more about situations that might impact the student or resident's behavior. Consider physiological factors, cultural factors, pharmacological factors, and life events. Physiological factors will include mental health issues, illnesses, genetic disorders, chronic conditions, and/or other types of impairments or difficulties. Cultural factors to be considered are social, responsive, behavioral, or influential differences between the respondent and the environment. Pharmacological factors would include any prescribed medication or treatment that is impacting the student's behavior. Finally, life event factors will encompass significant occurrences that might impact the student, such as a death, traumatic event, etc.

*Environmental Conditions* Environmental conditions involve the context or the circumstances in which the behavior occurs. This is the *who, what, when,* and *where* of the behavior. For instance, the *who* will involve people present, such as peers, teachers, parents, administrative staff, and/or paraprofessionals. The *what* will be the events or occurrence factors. This might be a little more difficult to identify. Some events could include curriculum being taught and actions being taken, such as transitioning, being asked to go to the board, or receiving a grade on an assignment. The *when* will include the time of day, such as morning, afternoon, a specific time, or even a specific season. The *where,* or setting, might include inside classroom, playground, office, cafeteria, hallway, and/or bathroom. Use the interview as a time to gain insight into contextual factors.

*Interventions* If a student or resident is exhibiting difficult behavior, most likely the people you are interviewing have attempted strategies to help improve the behavior. Some strategies might have been ineffective, and some might have been effective. It is important to gain an understanding of what has and has not worked. When it comes to behavior planning, this will be critical information to have gained.

*Function* The function of the behavior is the purpose it serves the respondent. It can be broken down into two purposes—to gain/obtain or to escape/avoid. The individuals you are interviewing will have opinions and ideas about the behavior they have seen and the purpose it might serve. Be sure to ask them so you can gain clarity on how they are viewing the student's behavior.

*Preferences* Understanding the student or resident's likes and dislikes can help you understand his or her current behavior. It can also help you to develop effective behavioral strategies. Personal preference inventories are highly recommended, especially in the planning phase of the FBA. However, the interview is an excellent time to ask about contextual preferences, tangible/reward preferences, and the types of people and personalities the student prefers. It is also an excellent time to find out contextual dislikes, items that are non-preferred, and personalities that the student struggles to be around.

Now that we have addressed the eight focus areas, let us talk about preparation. For some, this might seem more like a common sense model. But we believe that preparation is a part of professional responsibility.

Preparation for the interview consists of setting a positive atmosphere, identifying areas for clarification, and identifying an interview tool that works best for your situation. We promised you concrete information on setting the atmosphere. So, we will start there.

*Setting a Positive Atmosphere* Relationship building begins the first time you meet someone. In this moment, your behavior should be reassuring those you are interviewing that you will safeguard the information that will be shared. Whether this is the student, the staff, or the parents, this first contact should be both professional and respectful. When contacting the person for an interview, you need to establish the purpose of the interview and the time and date for the interview. Primarily, interviews are best completed face-to-face. However, if a person cannot adjust his or her schedule or is unable to come in, a phone interview can be scheduled. In the case of a language barrier or the need for an interpreter, it will be important to remain flexible as logistics are arranged to accommodate everyone's schedule.

During this initial contact, explain the purpose of the interview and the value of the information that you are gathering. Explain that the information will be used to develop an FBA and other behavior intervention planning. Also, explain who will be present at the interview and that the information gained will only be used to help the student. Information will be shared only with those who are necessary, such as treatment providers, educators, and caregivers. Access to this information is limited due to confidentiality.

Prior to the interview, make certain to have secured a private area to meet. On the day of the interview, arrive early and prepare the area. It never hurts to have some type of minimal refreshments, if only offering the interviewee a beverage. If you have never met the person you are interviewing, make certain to introduce yourself. During this introduction, explain how you became involved in the process, your role in the process, and allow the person you are interviewing a moment to ask you any questions before beginning the interview.

*Identifying Areas for Clarification* Prior to the interview, be sure to review any background information available to you. Any anecdotal information from teachers, notes from parents, disciplinary records, educational records, and medical history will be important. If the student has an Individualized Education Program (IEP), review this plan and all progress towards current goals. Take notes on any information that you need to clarify. For instance, if the student's records say that he takes medication, be sure to ask and determine if this medication has changed. It is important to have the most current information as possible.

*Identifying an Interview Tool*  After you have reviewed all the information about the student, you will have a clearer picture of his or her history and current behavioral difficulties. From all the information gathered including the target behavior, referral form, etc., you should have an idea of the types of questions you need to ask. In our experience, it is best to have a questionnaire or survey ready at the time of the interview. As noted previously, this book includes interview forms for the caregivers, staff, and the student. You might already work in an area that even has its own interview form. The important point here is to have your questions ready prior to the interview. If you have to add questions or change questions to suit the interview process, be prepared for this beforehand.

## Strategy Four: Application

With everything in place, the interview process should be much easier. To help you, we have a Interview Checklist in Appendix G.

> Drew and Michelle Wilding had been very cooperative. Gwen was pleased with all the information that she was getting from them. She had just asked about Willow's behavior. Michelle responded, "She just gets so out of control. It can be very difficult. She doesn't always seem mad. Just chaotic...."
> Gwen said, "I see. Michelle, can you tell me what 'out of control' looks like?"
> "Of course, Willow runs through the house. Sometimes she intentionally knocks over items, but sometimes it is not intentional. She tears up items, like our marriage license. She got into our important documents and would have torn up more paperwork if Drew hadn't caught her!"

## *Five Responses to Interview Challenges*

Once you have set the atmosphere and have chosen your assessment tool, it would be nice if you could simply execute the interview. Using the above tools and an appropriate questionnaire, you should be ready. Sometimes, however, there are challenges within the interview. To address those, we would like to add a few more suggestions.

*Clarify*  The staff or parent will often use generalized phrases. For example, when asking about target behaviors, a parent might say, "They get mad." Remember, you want them to tell you what the behavior looks like. You are trying to visualize the target behavior in a measurable way. An appropriate response to that statement might be a redirect. So, if this is what is said, redirect with, "What does mad look like?" You might add, "Does he hit other people or throw objects?"

*Rambling/Venting* Sometimes the interview can become an opportunity for the staff or parent to vent frustration. Or the staff or parent jump from one subject to the next and begin to talk about other events unrelated to the student. During these times, it is best to refocus the person gently. You might want to say, "I'm sure that is difficult. This interview will hopefully help to improve behavior. Let me ask you the next question." Or, "Let's see, I believe you were answering my question about...." Just remember to be respectful.

*Emotional* Sometimes the person you are interviewing can become very emotional. They might raise their voice or even begin to cry. This can be difficult, and navigating this situation appropriately is essential. Give the person a few moments, and perhaps offer understanding comfort, such as, "I know this is difficult and brings a lot of emotions to the surface." You should have a box of tissues available. Give the person a little time to regroup, and then gently redirect them back to the task.

*Unsafe* Although this has never occurred to either one of us, sometimes the person you are interviewing can become unsafe. When you are first seated, make certain that you have positioned yourself with no object between you and the door. In the event that the person you are interviewing becomes unsafe, leave the room and contact the nearest safety officer.

*Follow-Up* After the interview, you might realize you need more clarification or information. Be sure to let the interviewees know that you might have to do follow-up. They are generally very willing to talk with you again.

When interviewing the student, apply all of these principles. The only exception is that you need to interview the student *after* the observations.


## Strategy Five: What *Not* to Do

Hopefully, the interviews will be well executed and you will gain helpful information. However, we realize that there are many variables that are beyond your control. Here are six behaviors that you do not need to exhibit regarding interviews. If you do any of these six items, it could complicate the interviewing process and leave you with information gaps:

1. Do not be tardy or absent.
2. Do not become emotional. (Remain neutral and objective.)
3. Do not rush the interview.
4. Do not interview everyone. (Be selective. Too much data can be difficult to process.)
5. Do not interview the student before beginning observations.
6. Do not gossip about the interview.

## A Before-You-Proceed Checklist

1. Understand the importance of professionalism in the interview process.
2. Know the eight focus areas for an interview.
3. Explain how to set a positive atmosphere for an interview.
4. Execute the five responses to interview challenges.
5. List six behaviors to never exhibit regarding an interview.

**Author Takeaways**

*Takeaway from Stephanie, the behavior specialist:*

Interviewing can be challenging. Do not be hesitant. Sometimes asking the tougher questions or clarifying information is essential to the FBA process. Although you never want to pry, you should make certain that you have a clear understanding of the student's behavior. Sometimes that requires difficult questions. However, that is why building trust begins the first time you talk with the parents or staff. Professionalism and respect go a long way in building the type of interview dynamic that allows the interviewee to feel comfortable and secure in sharing information. A little more effort on the front end can save you a lot of effort during the interview.

*Takeaway from Alan, the school psychologist:*

Good interviewing skills take time to develop. After you complete your first several interviews, you will likely need to follow up and ask additional questions. Experience will help you to understand the most pertinent questions to ask. Interviewing can also be a delicate process with the parents. Although they are aware of the student's reported behaviors, they may not necessarily believe them ("I don't get it, he is perfectly fine at home."), they may blame the teacher ("Mrs. Johnson is always looking for the bad things he does. I'm not sure why she picks on him."), or they may become defensive ("My kid is fine. He is absolutely no different than any of the other kids his age. They'll all outgrow it."). These situations can be tough to deal with because it involves someone else's perceptions, but the point of interviewing is to collect the information you need in order to best help the student.

## References

Cipani, E., & Schock, K. M. (2010). *Functional behavioral assessment, diagnosis, and treatment: A complete system for education and mental health settings* (2nd ed.). New York: Springer.

Floyd, R. G., Phaneuf, R. L., & Wilczynski, S. M. (2005). Measurement properties of indirect assessment methods for functional behavioral assessment: A review of research. *School Psychology Review, 34*(1), 58–73.

Kinch, C., Lewis-Palmer, T., Hagan-Burke, S., & Sugai, G. (2001). A comparison of teacher and student functional behavior assessment interview information from low-risk and high-risk classrooms. *Education and Treatment of Children, 24*(4), 480–494.

Martella, R. C., Nelson, J. R., Marchand-Martella, N. E., & O'Reilly, M. (2012). *Comprehensive behavior management: Individualized, classroom, and schoolwide.* Thousand Oaks: Sage.

O'Neill, R. E., Horner, R. H., Ablin, R. W., Sprague, J. R., Storey, K., & Newton, J. S. (1996). Functional assessment and program development for problem behaviors: A practical handbook. New York: Brooks/Cole.

Umbreit, J., Ferro, J. B., Liaupsin, C. J., & Lane, K. L. (2006). *Functional behavioral assessment and function-based intervention: An effective, practical approach.* Upper Saddle River: Pearson.

# Chapter 7
# Process: Informal and Formal Assessments

## What You Need to Know

Data collection is ongoing through every stage of our multi-phasic approach. As we have moved through the Process phase, we have already begun to cover a range of appropriate ways to gather information. As we enter into this chapter, we introduce you to more. A full spectrum of assessments would include both informal and formal assessments, in addition to the interviews that we discussed in the last chapter. After conducting your interviews, you will have a better idea of a student's problematic behaviors. It is always a good idea to collect additional information through the use of informal and formal measures. Once you have the data from these assessments, you will analyze the data, which we will discuss in the next chapter. Formal measures are not necessary in the development of the functional behavioral assessment. However, understanding them will aid in records reviews and determining if the team should refer the student for more formal testing. Without a good understanding of all types of assessment, it would be difficult to navigate the options available. Unlike formal measures, informal measures do not require the assistance of a school psychologist, who must score and interpret the assessment. So, we will start with informal assessments.

## Strategy One: Understand the Basics

First things first: Let us define informal and formal assessments.

© Springer International Publishing Switzerland 2016                    71
S. M. Hadaway, A. W. Brue, *Practitioner's Guide to Functional Behavioral Assessment,*
Autism and Child Psychopathology Series, DOI 10.1007/978-3-319-23721-3_7

## *Informal Assessment*

### What Is It?

An informal assessment can include observations, interviews, and questionnaires. For the purposes of this chapter, let us focus our discussion on surveys and questionnaires so that we are not redundant with the content of other chapters. A *survey* is a process used to gather information, and it can involve a wide range of data collection methods, including a questionnaire. A *questionnaire,* meanwhile, is the actual instrument used to collect data from different individuals. Questionnaires can be completed on a classroom-, school-, or even district-wide basis. Administrators, teachers, and/or parents may complete them; you could also use a questionnaire to compare a student's perception of his own behaviors with that of other students when collecting information for an FBA.

## *Formal Assessment*

### What Is It?

A formal assessment includes standardized measures that allow you to compare one student's behavior to many other students (perhaps several thousand) of the same age—that is, *the standard.* These measures are usually developed by and purchased from one of the many test publishers who create different assessment measures. Formal assessments allow you to see which behaviors are not problematic, which ones are slightly problematic, and which ones are significantly problematic. Researchers have developed these measures in response to an increase in the number of FBAs being conducted in the school setting (Gable et al. 2014).

## Strategy Two: Understand the Scope

In the Process phase, we have been collecting data. As we continue to take you through this phase, we do want to make a few things clear regarding assessment. We will start with formal assessment. As briefly noted, a formal assessment is not necessary to the completion of an FBA. By mentioning them in this book, we want you to understand them. We are not trying to indicate that you must use them.

It is important to note that test publishers have certain restrictions about who can purchase, administer, score, and interpret these measures. Since many test publishers clearly define the parameters in which to use their measures, application is limited to qualified professionals. Many times, this would entail psychologists, psychological examiners, and diagnosticians. Within your organization, there are most likely individuals employed who are hired for the purpose of administering such measures, especially if you are in the public school system. If you come to believe that formal measures are needed for a student, it is best to work in conjunction with your school psychologist or organizational psychologist who can provide you with some guidance.

Even though you might not be able to administer a formal assessment, you will most likely come across them in records reviews. Primarily, we anticipate that you will see them in psychological evaluations located in eligibility reports for special education or brought in by the family. To help you with this, we have provided several assessments later on in this chapter to aid you with the familiarization process.

On the other hand, we would expect you to use informal assessments. In FBA, you will use informal assessments to gain information and group opinions. But you must be careful to understand that they are not concrete assessment measures. They are guides, not facts. They are, in essence, perceptions, and perceptions of behavior can vary widely; this is why information from multiple individuals is best practice. Informal assessments allow us to better understand the way in which others perceive the target behaviors.

## Strategy Three: What to Do

When using an informal assessment, the practitioner is responsible for an ethical administration of the instrument. There should be some type of protocol accompanying the measure. In the case of informal assessments, there might not be an accompanying protocol booklet, but there should still be some type of instructional guidance. In some cases, this might be as simple as directions. Despite the length of the guidance element, handling any measure consistently across administrations will strengthen the results.

Additionally, the practitioner is responsible for identifying the target behavior the instrument will measure. Prior to giving the informal assessment to someone, you need to determine the target behavior to be considered when responding to the assessment. Imagine that you are gathering information on two different target behaviors. One person responds to target behavior one on the informal measure you have given; the other person responds to target behavior two. When using informal assessments, there is a lot of value in identifying patterns of commonality, even if they are subjective. This is impossible if your returned assessments measure different target behaviors. Therefore, it is critical to make it clear which target behavior is considered on the informal assessment. If you want all target behaviors assessed, provide as many forms as needed for each behavior. On each form, clearly delineate which target behavior is being assessed.

Along with this, the practitioner is responsible for explaining the actual assessment. Do not assume that the person responding understands the format on the measure. Even if they are to only answer yes or no to the questions, be sure to go over the directions and make certain the person feels confident in the instructions. If the person responding is a poor reader or uncomfortable with completing the assessment independently, the practitioner can certainly read the assessment to the individual. Remember, these assessments are tools that can be used to support the interview data. Taking the time to make certain that they are understood is important.

Finally, the informal assessment is confidential. In order to maintain confidentiality, the practitioner should provide some type of privacy feature with the assessment, such as an envelope that can be sealed. This allows respondents to return the assessment without fear of their answers becoming public. As with all forms of data collection, the information gained from informal assessments is for the FBA and behavior planning. The information is not to be shared for other purposes and to personnel not directly involved in this process.

## Strategy Four: Application

There are many different types of informal assessments. We have chosen to detail the three that we have seen used within the school system: the *Functional Analysis Screening Tool*, the *Motivation Assessment Scale*, and the *Questions About Behavioral Function Scale*.

### *Functional Analysis Screening Tool (FAST)*

The *FAST* is a questionnaire used to identify factors that may influence the occurrence of problem behaviors. It is best if it is administered to several individuals—parents and teachers—who interact with the student on a regular basis. Results from the *FAST* should then be used as the basis for conducting direct observations in several different contexts to verify likely behavioral functions, clarify ambiguous functions, and identify other relevant factors that may not have been included in this instrument.

### *Motivation Assessment Scale (MAS)*

The *MAS* (Durand and Crimmins 1988) is a questionnaire that helps to identify situations in which a person is likely to behave a certain way. Once we have this information, we can make more informed decisions about the choice of appropriate rewards and support strategies. The *MAS* is a way in which to group information collected and perhaps gain a clearer understanding of everyone's opinion on the student's behaviors. This can be used in conjunction with formal assessment measures, which we will talk about next.

## *Questions About Behavioral Function (QABF)*

The *QABF* (Matson and Vollmer 1995) is a scale used to assess the function of maladaptive behaviors in persons who have been diagnosed with a developmental disability. This measure, typically completed by parents and caregivers, includes 25 items that ask a question about an individual's behavior. It is a Likert-type rating scale, and scores are obtained in five categories: attention, escape, physical, tangible, and nonsocial.

There are many measures that could be addressed when discussing formal assessments. After some consideration, we have decided to give you an overview of several formal assessment measures that may be used to collect data on a student's behavior. These are the measures that we see being used most often to assess general behavior problems, but there are many other measures available, including those designed to address more specific areas (e.g., anxiety, autism, depression). We will list some of those at the end of this chapter. Again, we want to note that test publishers have certain restrictions about who can purchase, administer, score, and interpret these measures. It is best to work in conjunction with your school psychologist who can provide you with some guidance.

## Achenbach System of Empirically Based Assessment (ASEBA)

The *ASEBA* offers a comprehensive approach to assess both adaptive and maladaptive functioning. It can be used with ages 1½–90+. The ASEBA includes different forms depending on the individual's age and who is completing it.

- Preschool Assessments
  - The *Preschool* forms cover the ages 1½–5 years. These forms obtain ratings from parents (Child Behavior Checklist) and day-care providers/teachers (Caregiver-Teacher Report Form) on 99 problem items. It also includes questions that allow the person completing it to write a description of the child's strengths and weaknesses. Standardized scores are obtained on the following scales:
    - Emotionally reactive
    - Anxious/depressed
    - Somatic complaints
    - Withdrawn
    - Sleep problems (Child Behavior Checklist only)
    - Attention problems
    - Aggressive behavior
    - Depressive problems

  - Anxiety problems
  - Autism spectrum problems
  - Attention-deficit/hyperactivity problems
  - Oppositional defiant problems
- School-Age Assessments
  - The *School-Age* forms cover the ages 6–18 years. These forms obtain ratings from parents (Child Behavior Checklist), teachers (Teacher's Report Form), and the student (Youth Self-Report); the student form is only for ages 11–18. Standardized scores are obtained on the following scales:
  - Anxious/depressed
  - Withdrawn/depressed
  - Somatic complaints
  - Social problems
  - Thought problems
  - Attention problems
  - Rule-breaking behavior
  - Aggressive behavior
  - Depressive problems
  - Anxiety problems
  - Attention-deficit/hyperactivity problems
  - Oppositional defiant problems
  - Conduct problems
- Adult Assessments
  - The *Adult* forms cover the ages 18–59 years. The two forms completed by adults are the Adult Self-Report (ASR) and Adult Behavior Checklist (ABCL). Standardized scores are obtained on the following scales:
  - Anxious/depressed
  - Withdrawn
  - Somatic complaints
  - Thought problems
  - Attention problems
  - Aggressive behavior
  - Rule-breaking behavior
  - Depressive problems
  - Anxiety problems
  - Avoidant personality problems
  - Attention-deficit/hyperactivity problems
  - Antisocial personality problems

In addition, these forms provide scores on:

  - Adaptive functioning (friends, spouse/partner, family, job, education, and personal strengths)
  - Substance use (tobacco, alcohol, and drugs)

# Behavior Assessment System for Children, Third Edition (BASC-3)

The *BASC-3* is a comprehensive set of rating scales and forms including three Teacher Rating Scales (TRS), three Parent Rating Scales (PRS), four Self-Report of Personality (SRP) forms, the Student Observation System (SOS), and the Structured Developmental History (SDH). The number of items ranges from 105 to 165 on the teacher forms, 139–175 on the parent forms, and 137–192 on the self-report forms. These scales are used to better understand the behaviors and emotions of children, adolescents, and young adults ages 2–21. Standardized scores are obtained on the following scales on the teacher and parent forms:

- Hyperactivity
- Aggression
- Conduct problems
- Anxiety
- Depression
- Somatization
- Attention problems
- Learning problems
- Atypicality
- Withdrawal
- Anger control
- Bullying
- Developmental social disorders
- Emotional self-control
- Executive functioning
- Negative emotionality
- Resiliency
- Activities of daily living
- Adaptability
- Social skills
- Leadership
- Study skills
- Functional communication

Standardized scores are obtained on the following scales on the child-, adolescent-, and/or college-age self-report forms (scales are applicable to all three forms unless otherwise noted):

- Attitude to school (child and adolescent)
- Attitude to teachers (child and adolescent)
- Sensation seeking (adolescent and college)
- Atypicality
- Locus of control
- Social stress

- Anxiety
- Depression
- Sense of inadequacy
- Somatization (adolescent and college)
- Attention problems
- Hyperactivity
- Alcohol abuse (college)
- Social maladjustment (college)
- Anger control (adolescent and college)
- Ego strength (adolescent and college)
- Mania (adolescent and college)
- Test anxiety (adolescent and college)
- Relations with parents
- Interpersonal relations
- Self-esteem
- Self-reliance

## Beck Youth Inventories, Second Edition (BYI-II)

The *BYI-II* is used to evaluate the emotional and social impairment in children and adolescents ages 7–18. There are five self-report inventories, which may be used individually or in different combinations. These five inventories each contain 20 questions about thoughts, feelings, and behaviors associated with emotional and social impairment. Standardized scores are obtained on the following scales:

- Depression inventory
- Anxiety inventory
- Anger inventory
- Disruptive behavior inventory
- Self-concept inventory

## Social Skills Improvement System Rating Scale (SSIS-RS)

The *SSIS-RS* helps to evaluate social skills, problem behaviors, and academic competence in students ages 3–18. There are forms for teachers (ages 8–12), parents (ages 8–12), and the student (ages 13–18), thus allowing for a comprehensive picture of social skills across school, home, and community settings. The number of items on the forms ranges from 75 to 83. Standardized scores are obtained on the following scales:

- Social skills: communication, cooperation, assertion, responsibility, empathy, engagement, self-control
- Competing problem behaviors: externalizing, bullying, hyperactivity/inattention, internalizing, autism spectrum
- Academic competence: reading achievement, math achievement, motivation to learn

## Conners Comprehensive Behavior Rating Scales (Conners CBRS)

The *Conners CBRS* rating scale is designed to provide a complete overview of child and adolescent concerns and disorders and assesses a wide spectrum of behaviors, emotions, and academic and social problems. The age range for this assessment is 6–18 for the parent and teacher forms and 8–18 for the self-report forms. There are 203 items on the parent form, 204 items on the teacher form, and 179 items on the self-report. Standardized scores are obtained on the following scales:

- Emotional distress
- Academic difficulties
- Separation fears
- Violence potential indicator
- Perfectionistic and compulsive behaviors
- Defiant/aggressive behaviors
- Hyperactivity/impulsivity
- Social problems
- Physical symptoms
- Attention-deficit/hyperactivity disorder (ADHD) hyperactive-impulsive
- ADHD inattentive
- ADHD combined
- Generalized anxiety disorder
- Conduct disorder
- Oppositional defiant disorder
- Manic episode
- Major depressive disorder
- Depressive episode, with mixed features
- Manic episode, with mixed features
- Separation anxiety disorder
- Social anxiety disorder
- Obsessive-compulsive disorder
- Autism spectrum disorder

## Burks Behavior Rating Scales, Second Edition (BBRS-2)

The *BBRS-2* helps to assess behavior problems in students ages 4–18. Forms are available for teachers and parents and include 100 items. Standardized scores are obtained on the following scales:

- Disruptive behavior
- Emotional problems
- Social withdrawal
- Ability deficits
- Physical deficits
- Weak self-confidence
- Attention and impulse control problems

The benefit of these formal measures is that they can be scored on a computer, which can yield some graphical representation of the scores. It makes it easy for the team to see the areas that are most problematic for the student. It may be especially helpful to parents who are having trouble understanding that their child's behavior is significantly different from that of other students of the same age. Scoring software is extra, but not necessary since the measures can be scored by hand.

The main drawback of formal measures is the cost involved in purchasing these tests. Test kits may be a couple of 100 dollars each, and additional forms must be purchased as they are used. If you are going to use formal measures, make sure that you have the money budgeted for their ongoing use.

## Formal Measures for Specific Problems

There are many other measures that the team may ask the school psychologist to use as part of the data collection process. We will list several of the measures here, but note that there are many more. These are the ones we see being used most frequently for the particular problem area.

### Assessing Anxiety
- Depression and Anxiety in Youth Scale (DAYS)
- Beck Anxiety Inventory (BAI)
- Beck Anxiety Inventory for Youth (BYI)
- Multidimensional Anxiety Scale for Children, Second Edition (MASC-2)
- Revised Children's Manifest Anxiety Scale, Second Edition (RCMAS-2)
- Social Phobia and Anxiety Inventory for Children (SPAI-C)
- Spence Children's Anxiety Scale (SCAS)
- *State-Trait Anxiety Inventory for Children (STAIC)*

### Assessing Attention/Hyperactivity/Impulsivity
- ADHD Rating Scale-IV (ADHD-IV)
- Attention Deficit Disorders Evaluation Scale, Fourth Edition (ADDES-4)

- Barkley Adult ADHD Rating Scale-IV (BAARS-IV)
- *Conners, Third Edition (Conners 3)*

**Assessing Autism**
- Asperger Syndrome Diagnostic Scale (ASDS)
- Autism Diagnostic Interview—Revised (ADI-R)
- Autism Diagnostic Observation Schedules, Second Edition (ADOS-2)
- Childhood Autism Rating Scale, Second Edition (CARS-2)
- Gilliam Asperger's Disorder Scale (GADS)
- Gilliam Autism Rating Scale, Third Edition (GARS-3)
- *Krug Asperger's Disorder Index (KADI)*

**Assessing Depression**
- Children's Depression Inventory, Second Edition (CDI-2)
- Children's Depression Rating Scale—Revised (CDRS-R)
- Depression and Anxiety in Youth Scale (DAYS)
- Reynolds Adolescent Depression Scale, Second Edition (RADS-2)
- *Reynolds Child Depression Scale, Second Edition (RCDS-2)*

> Back at Good Hope Elementary, Gwen Gillespie was scoring the FAST measures she had received back from the staff and Mr. and Mrs. Wilding.
> She was going through the rankings. "Well," she said aloud, "This is interesting! Look at how they each ranked Escape/Avoidance...."
> Without realizing it, she helped herself to her fourth piece of chocolate.

# A Before-You-Proceed Checklist

1. Understand the difference between formal assessments and informal assessments.
2. Name three characteristics of formal assessments.
3. Name three responsibilities involved in informal assessments.
4. Review the lists of informal and formal assessments.

**Author Takeaways**
*Takeaway from Stephanie, the behavior specialist:*
    Assessment is a benefit to the FBA process. It provides valuable information regarding the individual's abilities, skills, and personality features. Informal assessments allow the practitioner to gain insight into the perceptions of both caregivers and professionals regarding the behavior of the student. Although subjective, the information related in the assessment process will inform the practitioner. Linked with records, interviews, and observations, patterns will begin to emerge. Just as with interviews, there may be times where you need to ask follow-up questions. That is fine! Remember, it is okay to ask for clarification.

*Takeaway from Alan, the school psychologist:*
There are many different tools that can be used to collect information about a student and his or her behavior. Informal and formal measures may be used individually or in combination; we suggest a comprehensive, combination approach. While formal measures will cost money, their use can be very beneficial when you need to demonstrate that a student's behavior is problematic compared to other students of the same age. When used in conjunction with interviews, you should have collected enough information from informal and formal measures to begin the data analysis process.

# References

Durand, V. M., & Crimmins, D. B. (1988). Identifying the variables maintaining self-injurious behavior. *Journal of Autism and Developmental Disorders, 18*(1), 99–117.
Gable, R. A., Park, K. L., & Scott, T. M. (2014). Functional behavioral assessment and students at risk for or with emotional disabilities: Current issues and considerations. *Education and Treatment of Children, 37*(1), 111–135.
Matson, J. L., & Vollmer, T. (1995). *User's guide: Questions about behavioral function (QABF).* Baton Rouge: Scientific Publishers.

# Chapter 8
# Process: Observation

## What You Need to Know

Until now, we have mainly discussed gaining information from secondary sources. Within this chapter, we complete our guidance through phase one, *Process*. As
noted, Process is the beginning phase of functional behavioral assessment (FBA).
This phase precedes analysis by providing data to inform further decision-making.
When successfully practiced, it moves the practitioner into determining the purpose
of the exhibited behavior.

Data collection can be gathered both indirectly and directly. As we move away
from indirect methods of data collecting, we will begin our discussion of direct observation. Direct observation is not just about watching a student; it requires knowledge of data collection methods and an understanding of when to use these methods. As a point of distinction, this book is guiding the reader to the development
of an FBA. We have noted that functional behavioral analysis may or may not be a
part of this process. When conducting a functional behavioral analysis, a third type
of data collection called experimental observational data is used. The functional behavioral analysis tests the hypothesis for the target behavior by manipulating a variable to determine if a behavior is reinforced. For the purposes presented here, direct
observational data will *not* involve interjecting the observer into the experience of
the student. Given these guidelines, the classroom or naturalized setting observation
needs to remain independent of observer participation. A portion of this chapter will
be dedicated to observer conduct.

## Strategy One: Understand the Basics

Data collection is a systematic process to collect information. In the case of an
FBA, the information gathered is on the identified target behavior. Over the last few
chapters, you have learned about secondary sources of information such as records,
interviews, and informal assessments. These secondary sources represent indirect
observational data.

© Springer International Publishing Switzerland 2016                                    83
S. M. Hadaway, A. W. Brue, *Practitioner's Guide to Functional Behavioral Assessment,*
Autism and Child Psychopathology Series, DOI 10.1007/978-3-319-23721-3_8

Direct observational data is the information you gather. It is the firsthand recordings of the student or resident's behavior derived from observation. Although indirect observational data gives you access to the viewpoints of others, it is by nature, subjective. Even though this might be valuable information to garner, it remains perspective driven. Within the FBA, it becomes necessary to look beyond the subjective into the objective features of behavior. You might recognize these objective features by identifiers such as frequency, duration, and intensity. Direct observational data allows you to collect this data by means of recording methods (Gresham et al. 2001).

If you can think back to general psychology, you might remember reading about the Hawthorne effect. The Hawthorne effect indicates that subjects who are being observed will demonstrate a change in their behavior based on the observation being conducted. Although studying the impact of an observer on a subject's behavior is not our focus, it is important to understand that adding a person to a setting will impact the setting. And, in turn, it will most likely impact the target behavior. Therefore, it is important when attempting an observation in a classroom or residential setting that the observer's conduct remains professional and appropriate for the situation.

## Five Recommendations for Observer Conduct

*Preparation* One of the methods to facilitate a successful observation is preparation. First things first, let someone know you will be coming. Prior to beginning an observation, be sure to talk with the adults who will be present during the observation. If the environment is one in which the observer will be noticed when present, it is important to minimize this interruption. If you have ever observed in a classroom, you know that students will be very curious about this "stranger" in the room. They often want to know who you are, why you are there, or if you are someone's mother or father. All of the questions they pose are to be expected. You are a new person coming into their learning environment. You can minimize this impact by allowing the adult in charge to remain in charge. If you enter a classroom and one or more questions are asked about your presence, allow the adult in charge to answer. It might be best for the adult in charge to just say that you will be coming in from time to time for observation and everyone should continue as normal when you arrive. Do not leave any of this to chance. Prior to your observation, discuss these eventualities with staff members.

Second, *never* explain that you are there to observe a specific student or resident. Prior to your observation, all adults involved should understand that they should avoid phrases like, "He has been awful today!" or "That's her sitting right there." The adults in the room should not point out the student/resident or talk to you about his or her behavior in front of him/her or any peers. Prior to your arrival, you should know either where the student/resident sits or work out a discreet way that you can be shown who the individual is without everyone in the room knowing. If the adults in the setting need to tell you about a behavior, it should be done outside of the direct observation. This is critical to both your objectivity and reducing the impact of your presence in the environment.

*Professionalism* We are aware that we have covered professional conduct, but it remains an important part of your effectiveness during direct observation. So, just to recap, when entering the setting, it is important to conduct yourself with the policies that govern the environment. Dress code, language, and behavior are marks of professionalism. Your behavior should exemplify a standard of behavior that the institution you are working in would uphold.

*Focus* It is difficult to gather data when your attention is divided. To help with your focus, avoid interjecting yourself into the lesson, tasks or activities in the classroom or treatment environment. Certainly, in a room full of students/residents, one or two might talk to you. Be mindful of what is happening in the environment. Redirect any individual talking to you back to the adults present in the room. If a student/resident you are not observing requests your assistance, refer them back to the adult in charge.

*Positioning* Sometimes finding the right place to stand or sit is difficult in a crowded room. It is usually best to position yourself at the back or to the side of a room with the individual you are observing in your line of sight. Avoid following the student/resident around. If the class or group lines up for a bathroom break, you could follow them into the hall and stand with another adult or further away from the group. If the individual you are observing goes alone to the restroom, to the office, or on another short errand, it is best to just note the time that he or she was out of class. You do not want to follow the student/resident from place to place. This makes it clear that you are there to observe him/her.

*Confidentiality* By now, you have read about confidentiality multiple times in this book. We hope that underscores the importance of maintaining confidentiality. The events that you observe should be treated with confidentiality. If another teacher, counselor, parent, or an office worker attempts to talk to you about the student or resident's behavior, it is best to redirect them to the primary teacher. The events you observe and have privy to are not for gossip in the hallway.

## *Four Guidelines for Successful Observations*

*Objectivity* First, the observations need to remain objective. As noted previously, direct observational data comes from primary observations. It is the information gleaned from direct student observation. Although the student's teacher or other staff members might see the student or subject daily, direct observational data is most beneficial when it is gathered by an objective person. Within a team approach, this could be the lead special education teacher, a different teacher, the school psychologist, the school counselor, or any other professional who is part of the student's team. If a specialist is conducting the FBA, he/she will gather this information.

*Accuracy* Second, make certain the data is accurate. An individual's goals, interventions, successes, and failures will be derived and measured by data collection. There is no strategy or plan that will be significantly effective based on inaccurate data. A person's progress will never be adequately identified based on inaccurate data. It is not enough to collect data; it needs to be accurately collected. Otherwise, the fidelity of both progress and programming are compromised, and some research has questioned whether school personnel can conduct FBAs with enough fidelity to result in students' behavior change (e.g., Cone 1997; Crone et al. 2007; Gresham et al. 1999).

*Meaningfulness* Third, insure the data you are collecting is meaningful. Anyone can observe a subject and collect data. You can collect data on how many times someone blinks, how many times someone erases an answer, or how many times someone asks to change seats. Certainly, there is information to be gleaned from this data. In the development of FBA, the focus should be on the *target behavior* and the events surrounding the occurrence of the target behavior. So, it is not necessary to identify every single behavior a subject exhibits. Rather, identify the meaningful data that applies to the target behavior.

Additionally, be aware of behaviors that have not been identified but are atypical, inappropriate, interfering, uncontrolled, and dangerous. We have both observed students with an interfering behavior that was actually more severe than the target behavior named. If this happens, collect data on this unidentified behavior. This information might supersede the original target behaviors because of the frequency or seriousness of the behavior. These behaviors might cluster with identified behaviors illuminating a different function than first identified (Scott et al. 2005). Either way, this is meaningful information that should be delivered to the team for consideration.

*Timeliness* Finally, data collection should be timely. When gathering information for an FBA, the data need to be timely. Old data might give us historical information and a way to measure improvement or lack of improvement, but we are looking for recent data. A lot can change in an individual's life over the passage of time. Those events can alter the fidelity of the data impacting the function of the student or resident's behavior. Data collection is a key component to the development of an FBA. It should be gathered during the FBA process.

## Strategy Two: Understand the Scope

There are two questions that we constantly hear when advising practitioners on direct observation. One question is, "How many times do I have to observe the student?" The other is, "How long do I observe the student?" We are going to take a moment and answer these two questions and a few others regarding direct observation.

How many times does a practitioner need to observe a student's behavior? On the surface, that might seem like a simple question, but it really is not. Our general rule is to observe the student long enough to obtain sufficient data. For us, we tend to believe that more is better. In the case of severe behavior, it is not uncommon for us to observe a student over ten times. Typically, we suggest that you observe 5–10 times, usually leaning towards more rather than less. There can be many different variables, so it is important to gain an understanding of how the student's behavior is affected by the environment.

How long is an observation? That depends on whether you are observing a specific activity, an event, a group, or a class. It is preferable to gather information about behavior exhibited during a range of activities or events. This gives you a truer picture of the behavior that you are observing. Even though we have heard of very brief observations, it is our hope that your observations will last a minimum of 30 min. In our practice, we do not typically observe a student all day long. It seems to us that following a student from place to place impacts the environment and the student significantly. We attempt to observe anywhere between 30 and 120 min, depending on the situation, severity, and needs involved.

Should an observation take place in only one setting? That depends, I (Stephanie) once observed a student only when the school had a fire drill since this was the only time a particular behavior occurred. Through a series of desensitization strategies, the student had successfully eliminated tantrum behavior associated with loud noises, except during a fire drill. So I observed the student during every fire drill. Having said that, we believe that is the exception rather than the rule.

Observing a student across a range of settings allows the observer to gain a clearer understanding of day-to-day functioning. For example, a student has verbally aggressive behavior in reading. Even if this behavior has never occurred in math class, it is important to see what is different in math class than in reading. Observation allows the practitioner to see the behavior or the lack of behavior across a variety of environments.

What if the target behavior does not occur? There are several times that the target behavior does not emerge during an observation. We have both stood and listened to exasperated administrators, counselors, and teachers reassure us that the behavior does occur. We believe them. One advantage to multiple observations is that given certain environmental conditions, a learned behavior will occur. We just have to be present. Just give it time. If for some reason it never occurs, it might be time to take note of environmental factors and reconsider what is and is not reinforcing the behavior. One last note—there are many individuals whose behavior improves in the presence of an observer. Most of the time, it has been our experience that if we observe long enough, this type of individual will eventually become familiar with our presence, and the target behavior will reemerge.

Okay, so how do you collect the data? That is a very good question. It depends on the behavior. The most common forms we use are the antecedent-behavior-consequence (ABC) chart and the scatterplot, but there are many ways to collect data. In order to choose the right instrument, we have provided some additional information on types of data collection for you.

## Strategy Three: What to Do

There are different ways in which direct observational data can be collected. Choosing the most efficient way depends on the behavior that is being observed. Baseline data is the first set of data; all future progress will be measured against the baseline data (Lane et al. 2015). For instance, Bobby talks out 25 times during an hour-long math lesson. As goals and strategies are implemented, it is hoped that Bobby would talk out fewer times. After 2 weeks of intervention, Bobby's talking out would be measured again. To determine if improvement has been made, the 25 times of talking out would be the data to which everything else is measured and compared.

## *Data Collection Methods*

**Event Recording** This is a method of data collection documenting the number of times a behavior occurs in a specified time period. To use this method, the observer might make a tally mark on a recording sheet, mark through a number on a recording sheet, drop a token into a jar, use a click counter, or even place a sticker on a sheet of paper. The major advantage of event recording is that it is easily accessible to even a busy teacher.

- *Frequency Collection*—Utilize this method when the length of observation is the same from day to day. Simply count the number of times the student is engaged in the targeted behavior. At the end of the time period, you have the frequency of the behavior. For instance, Tessa talks out 60 times during a 30-min reading lesson. Every time Tessa talks out during the observation period, a tally mark is placed on the recording sheet.
- *Rate*—Utilize this method when the length of observation time varies from day to day. Count the number of times the student engaged in the targeted behavior, then divide the engagement amount by the length of time the behavior occurred. For instance, Tessa talks out 60 times during a 30-min reading lesson. Tomorrow, she will be observed in an hour-long math segment. So, frequency data is not appropriate.
  - Calculate rate by dividing 60 by 30: $60/30 = 2$. Tessa talked out two times per minute in her reading lesson.

Event recording is best used when:

- The behavior does not occur with a high rate of frequency (e.g., tapping foot or talking with friends).
- The behavior has a clear beginning and end (e.g., temper tantrum).
- Limited staff to record data.
- It is important to know the amount of time a behavior occurs.

**Interval Recording** This is a method of data collection documenting the occurrence or lack of occurrence of the target behavior in a specified time interval. Instead of recording every occurrence, the observer records the target behavior data at preselected, equal time intervals and denotes whether the behavior is occurring. For instance, 60 min might be divided into twelve 5-min time intervals. When using interval recording, it is necessary to have some type of timing device, such as a timer or stopwatch. It is also good to have an auditory reminder, such as a timer beep, to keep track of intervals.

- *Partial-interval recording*—Utilize this method when the actual time of occurrence of the target behavior is important and the intention of data collection is behavior reduction. This method is also used when event recording is not feasible. For instance, if there is a high rate of behavior, the behavior occurs quickly or the behavior occurs constantly and/or the behavior does not have a clear beginning and end. To collect the data, use a recording sheet with the preselected time intervals. At the selected time, note the student and determine if the target behavior occurs during the interval. Then, mark the sheet with an "X" or "0," Yes or No, or a plus or minus sign. You do not record if the behavior occurs more than one time in an interval. If the behavior is occurring frequently, this can be a time saver because once the behavior is noted, the recording is finished until the next interval. Since partial-interval recording is an estimate, keep the time interval small. Certainly, a 10-min time interval is the longest period suggested. For example, Tessa talks out frequently in class. She is observed for 30 min in 3-min intervals; this gives you ten intervals. During observation, Tessa talked out during seven intervals. To calculate, take the number of intervals Tessa talked out and divide it by the total number of intervals observed. Then, multiply by 100.
  - $7/10 = 0.70$, $0.70 \times 100 = 70\%$. Tessa talked out 70 % of the observed time.
- *Whole-interval recording*—Utilize this method when you want to estimate the duration of a target behavior and you want to increase a behavior. This method is also used when event recording is not feasible. For instance, there is a high rate of behavior and/or the behavior does not have a clear beginning and end. The primary difference between whole-interval recording and partial-interval recording is that in whole-interval recording, the target behavior must occur for the *entire* interval before it is marked. To collect the data, use a recording sheet with the preselected time intervals. At the selected time, observe the student and determine if the target behavior occurs throughout the interval. Then, mark the sheet with an "X" or "0," Yes or No, or a plus or minus sign. As with partial-interval recording, keep the time interval small. Again, a 10-min time interval is the longest period suggested. The calculation for both whole-interval recording and partial-interval recording is the same. For example, Tessa talks out frequently in class. She is observed for 30 min in 3-min intervals; this gives you ten intervals. During observation, Tessa talked out during seven intervals. To calculate, take the number of intervals Tessa talked out and divide it by the total number of intervals observed. Then, multiply by 100.
  - $7/10 = 0.70$, $0.70 \times 100 = 70\%$. Tessa talked out 70 % of the observed time.

Whole-interval recording is a time-consuming process. It requires at least two people present to complete the observations.

- *Scatterplot*—Utilize this method when you want to know the time of day a behavior occurs. Although it will not provide antecedent or consequent data, a scatterplot will indicate trends or patterns as to the contextual factors involved with the targeted behavior. To collect this type of data, the observer uses a special data sheet, a scatterplot. The scatterplot is actually a grid with the vertical line divided into periods of time. The periods of time are determined by the observer and the type of activity or interval that is needed. The horizontal line contains the date. Now, there are a wide range of scatterplots. They can range from very simple to very complex. Some include a code which indicates the type of behavior that was observed. During the provided intervals, you write the appropriate code down. Others might indicate what the individual was doing or what activity was taking place during the interval of occurrence. Below, there is an example of a simple scatterplot.

**Scatter Plot**

Name: _____        Target Behavior: _____

Setting: _____

| Time | Monday Date: | Tuesday Date: | Wednesday Date: | Thursday Date: | Friday Date: |
|---|---|---|---|---|---|
| 8:00-8:30 | | | | | |
| 8:30-9:00 | | | | | |
| 9:00-9:30 | | | | | |
| 9:30-10:00 | | | | | |
| 10:00-10:30 | | | | | |
| 10:30-11:00 | | | | | |

Additionally, scatterplots are usually reported as the percentage of intervals in which the behavior occurred.

For example, Tessa talks out in seven intervals over a period of ten intervals.

- $7/10 = 0.70$.
- $0.70 \times 100 = 70\%$.
- Tessa talked out 70% of intervals on (include the date).

Interval recording is best used when:

- The behavior occurs with a high rate of frequency (e.g., tapping foot or talking with friends).
- The behavior does not have a clear beginning and end (e.g., temper tantrum).
- Access to experienced and additional staff. (The scatterplot does not require additional staff.)

**Duration Recording** This is a method of data collection documenting how long a behavior occurs. Duration recording will record the total time or percentage of time that a behavior occurs within a specified time period. Behavior is measured from the time it begins until the time it stops. A stopwatch is a necessity, especially if it is essential to measure time in seconds. Duration recording can be used to target an increase or decrease in behavior. For example, Tessa talked out conversationally three times in her 30-min math lesson. Each lasted a different length of time—4, 3, and 5 min—for a total duration of 12 min during the 30-min math lesson.

- Percentage of observation with the behavior:
  $12/30$ min $= 0.40$
  $0.40 \times 100 = 40\%$
  Tessa's talking occurred during 40 % of the observation.
- Average duration of talking out behavior:
  12 min/3 talking-out episodes = an average of 4 min per talking-out episodes.

Duration recording is best used when:

- The length of the behavior is the focus of the observation.
- The behavior does have a clear beginning and end (e.g., temper tantrum).
- The behavior occurs over a period of time, not in quick succession or rapidly.

**Latency Recording** This is a method of data collection documenting the length of elapsed time between the onset of a stimulus and the occurrence of a particular behavior. Latency recording can be used when you want to decrease the amount of time it takes for a student to respond to a specific instruction (e.g., how long he/she takes to begin an assignment after being provided with the verbal instructions) or other stimulus (e.g., providing a verbal response after being asked a question). A stopwatch can be used to measure the length of time between the presentation of the stimulus and the start of the desired behavior.

For example, Tessa talked out three times conversationally during her 30-min math lesson. Her teacher prompted her with a verbal reminder to begin her work each time. Tessa did not immediately return to her work. Tessa took 3 min (180 s), 2 min (120 s), and 1 min (60 s) to begin her work.

- $3 + 2 + 1 = 6$.
- $6/3 = 2$.
- Tessa took an average of 2 min to start her math assignment.

If you have smaller units of time, you can calculate the seconds it took Tessa to begin her math assignment.

Latency recording is best used when:

- The length of time it takes the individual to begin the expected behavior is needed.
- The behavior does have a clear beginning and end.
- The behavior is not ongoing.
- The behavior does not occur in quick succession or rapidly.

Prior to discussing ABC data collection, we want to emphasize the importance of descriptive analysis. Martella et al. (2012) indicate that, "Descriptive analyses involve the direct observation of the student in the natural environment where the challenging behavior is most likely to occur. Descriptive analyses can take several forms, such as ABC analyses, observation forms, and scatter plots" (p. 124). We hope by this point, you are familiar with the ABC acronym and how it relates to the FBA process. It is important that you understand and know how to use this type of data collection form. In reality, the form is not complicated to use, but your objectivity and close observation of the events during observation are necessary for successful analysis.

## *ABC Data Collection*

This is a method of descriptive analysis that allows the observer to document the environmental variables related to the target behavior. To use this method, the observer fills out a three-column form that identifies the target behavior and the contextual factors occurring in the environment. These contextual factors include the antecedent information (what comes before) and the consequent information (what comes after). The behavior, which goes in the middle column, is the act or action that the individual exhibits. There are many variations of this form, but all will have the ABC format in common. The benefit to using ABC data collection is that it identifies the events and happenings occurring in and around the student or resident's behavior.

ABC data recording is best used when:

- An FBA is being completed.
- Additional personnel are available.
- The observer has an ample amount of time to record events.

So, let's dig a little deeper with ABC data collection.

## Strategy Four: Application

We enter into any FBA discussion with the assumption that behavior is learned. The three-term contingency model explains how behavior is elicited by the environment and how the consequences of behavior can affect the future occurrence of behavior. The basic premise of an FBA is that through a series of methods, one can determine the relationship between two events—a behavior and a consequence. When the impact is studied and understood, a functional relationship can be identified between the two.

Here is a quick reminder:

*Antecedent*—This is the preceding stimulus. It is the event, experience, or circumstance that happened just before the behavior *(what comes before)*. It is sometimes called a fast trigger.

*Behavior*—This is the target behavior. It is the act or action that the student or client exhibited.

*Consequence*—This is the event, experience, or circumstance that happened right after the behavior *(what comes after)*.

When completing an FBA you must understand how to gather data using an ABC form. So, what do you do?

A (antecedent)-**B** (behavior)-**C** (consequence) data collection is about identifying the contextual variables that precede and follow a target behavior. It is a form of data collection requiring the observer to record what happens before the target behavior, during the target behavior, and after the target behavior.

So, let us practice just that. Earlier in this book, we used a set of examples to identify target behaviors. Here, we will use those same examples to practice identifying ABC.

## *Refusals*

Mark refuses to work in math class. Today he was given an assignment. When his teacher verbally prompted him to work, Mark yelled, "No." He was sent into the hallway for being disrespectful.

Antecedent: Mark's teacher verbally prompts him to do his math assignment.
Behavior: Mark yells, "No."
Consequence: Mark is sent into the hallway.

## *Physical Aggressive*

Ava is playing a game with another student. She loses the game. Ava turns and punches the other student in the arm, causing an instant bruise. Ava is reprimanded by her teacher and given a disciplinary referral to the office.

Antecedent: Ava loses a game she is playing with another student.
Behavior: Ava punches the other student in the arm leaving a bruise.
Consequence: Ava's teacher verbally reprimands her and sends her to the office with a discipline referral.

## *Out-of-Area Behavior*

Juan appears very restless. He will remain in his seat during individual assignments. However, when placed in a group, he often leaves his seat. He will wander throughout the room, sometimes running and skipping. Juan is redirected to his seat by his teacher and allowed to work independently at his desk.

Antecedent: Juan is placed in a group.
Behavior: Juan leaves his seat, running and skipping around the room.
Consequence: Juan is redirected to his seat by his teacher and allowed to work in-
dependently at his desk.

## *Disruptive*

Carla does not like to read. Every time her class begins to read, Carla starts talking
out to the teacher. Today, she is talking about going to the movies. Reading instruction is delayed. Carla's teacher verbally warns her explaining that if her behavior
continues she will not earn a token at the end of reading instruction.

Antecedent: The class begins to read.
Behavior: Carla talks out about going to the movies.
Consequence: Reading is delayed, and Carla's teacher verbally warns her that she
will not earn a token if her behavior continues.

Here is another example: Mitch leaves his seat and runs around the classroom.
His target behavior is, "Mitch leaves his assigned area in the classroom without
permission."

| Antecedent | Behavior | Consequence |
|---|---|---|
| Teacher asks all students to come to the calendar area | Mitch gets up and begins running around the classroom | Teacher verbally redirects Mitch to come to the calendar area and sit down |
| The entire class has made it to the calendar area. The teacher asks Mitch again to come and join the rest of the class | Mitch laughs and continues to run around the room | Two students tell Mitch to hurry up and sit down |
| Teacher verbally warns Mitch that if he does not sit down, he will change his color | Mitch pauses but then begins to run around the room again | Teacher moves Mitch's color from green to yellow |
| Teacher walks over and moves Mitch's color on the student chart from green to yellow | Mitch pauses and yells, "No" | Teacher verbally redirects him to sit down with his peers |
| Teacher verbally warns Mitch that she will change his color to red if he does not sit down | Mitch begins to cry but joins the group at the calendar area | Teacher praises him and tells him he can earn going back to green if he makes good choices the rest of the day |

When using an ABC form, it will be important to note the time and student name on
the form. We have included an ABC Data Collection Sheet in Appendix H.

> Gwen Gillespie had enjoyed observing Willow Wilding. She was quite an artist! Unfortu-
> nately, so much of this was not appreciated because of her behavior. Gwen remembered
> what Michelle had said about her daughter. Her behavioral description had been "out of
> control." Gwen could easily see why this phrase had entered Mrs. Wilding's mind.
> Gwen gathered her last ABC Chart and headed from the room. It was finally time to analyze
> the data.

It is at this point that we conclude the Willow Wilding vignettes in the book. As mentioned, Willow's FBA and behavior intervention plan can be found in Chap. 12.

## Strategy Five: What Not to Do

Here are things to avoid:

1. Do not misuse or mischaracterize the data.
2. Do not allow your own biases and values to cloud your judgment.
3. Do not interrupt or intrude in the environment where you are observing.
4. Do not rush an observation.
5. Do not leave this chapter without understanding data collection methods.

## A Before-You-Proceed Checklist

1. Familiarize yourself with the five recommendations for observer conduct.
2. Know the four guidelines for successful observation.
3. Understand how long an observation should last.
4. Understand the difference between event recording, interval recording, duration recording, and latency recording.
5. Understand the term scatterplot.
6. Know how to conduct ABC data collection.

**Author Takeaways**

*Takeaway from Stephanie, the behavioral specialist:*

Prior to any observation, I always talk to the staff about my expectations regarding their behavior when I am observing in a classroom. It is very tempting for staff struggling with a student's behavior to point it out when I walk into a room. I cannot underscore enough how much that impacts the objectivity of the observation. Always prepare the school, treatment center, or residential program for your visit. Let them know that talking about the individual in front of him/her or other people is problematic to the FBA process. Communicating beforehand might not eliminate all of this behavior, but it will help.

*Takeaway from Alan, the school psychologist:*

As we discussed elsewhere, detailed information is necessary in order to plan for the FBA. You need as many details as possible so that you can choose the most appropriate data collection method. As a school psychologist, I know that my approach is much different if I need to record the number of behaviors versus the length of a particular behavior. For example, if I am recording the number of behaviors and the behavior occurs much more frequently in the afternoon, then I will plan to do my observations in the afternoon. In this way, I know that I am identifying the behavior at its worst, with an understanding that at other times of day, the behavior may not be viewed as being so problematic.

# References

Cone, J. D. (1997). Issues in functional analysis in behavioral assessment. *Behaviour Research and Therapy, 35*(3), 259–275.

Crone, D. A., Hawken, L. S., & Bergtstrom, M. K. (2007). A demonstration of training, implementing and using functional assessment in 10 elementary and middle school settings. *Journal of Positive Behavior Intervention, 9*(1), 15–29.

Gresham, F. M., Quinn, M. M., & Restori, A. (1999). Methodological issues in functional analysis: Generalizability to other disability groups. *Behavioral Disorders, 24*(2), 180–182.

Gresham, F. M., Watson, T. S., & Skinner, C. H. (2001). Functional behavioral assessment: Principles, procedures, and future directions. *School Psychology Review, 30*(2), 156–172.

Lane, K. L., Oakes, W. P., Powers, L., Diebold, T., Germer, K., Common, E. A., & Brunsting (2015). Improving teachers' knowledge of functional assessment-based interventions: Outcomes of a professional development series. *Education and Treatment of Children, 38*(1), 93–120.

Martella, R. C., Nelson, J. R., Marchand-Martella, N. E., & O'Reilly, M. (2012). *Comprehensive behavior management: Individualized, classroom, and schoolwide*. Thousand Oaks: Sage.

Scott, T. M., Liaupsin, C., Nelson, C. M., & McIntyre (2005). Team-based functional behavior assessment as a proactive public school process: A descriptive analysis of current barriers. *Journal of Behavioral Education, 14*(1), 57–71.

# Part III
# Phase II: Purpose

*Purpose* is the second phase of functional behavioral assessment.

**Professional Responsibilities** Within *Purpose,* the practitioner would organize the data, analyze the data, and formulate the hypothesis statement.

**Alternative View** The *Purpose* phase could also be considered the *analysis and formulation phase.* This phase is about organizing, reflecting, and analyzing.

**Task List** The practitioner will complete or lead a team in completing the following list:

1. Organize data
2. Graph data
3. Analyze data
4. Formulate hypothesis

**Goal** By the end of this phase, the practitioner will have used reliable data to form a hypothesis statement regarding the function of the target behavior(s).

# Chapter 9
# Purpose: Analysis of the Data

## What You Need to Know

Until now, the bulk of this book has been spent in what we have termed *Process,* or the working phase. At this stage in the functional behavioral assessment (FBA) approach, you have collected data from four distinct sources: records, interviews, informal assessments, and your own observational data. You have completed the tasks that were prescribed in Phase I, and you are standing on the precipice of the next phase, *Purpose.*

Within Purpose, the practitioner begins data analysis. This involves looking critically at all of the information gathered. It is a detail-oriented task that requires organization and reflection. Analysis ushers the practitioner forward into the development of the hypothesis statement. But remember, if the data analysis is weak, the hypothesis will be weak. Therefore, we will approach this task carefully and with diligence.

So, let us start with the fundamentals.

## *Strategy One: Understand the Basics*

There are two different types of data. Quantitative data are numerically based; it is the information that uses numbers. Identifying the frequency of an outburst or the duration of an outburst is quantitative in nature. It relies on precise measurement and is objective. The other type of data is qualitative. Qualitative data is the information that is derived from interviews or reviewing someone's anecdotal notes. It can sometimes be open-ended, and it is subjective (Johnson and Christensen 2008; Lichtman 2006).

© Springer International Publishing Switzerland 2016

S. M. Hadaway, A. W. Brue, *Practitioner's Guide to Functional Behavioral Assessment,*
Autism and Child Psychopathology Series, DOI 10.1007/978-3-319-23721-3_9

## *Strategy Two: Understand the Scope*

Up to this point, you have been busy developing an FBA. You have gathered information from many sources. But, what have you actually been doing? What has been the point of all the tasks you have undertaken? What has been your goal? If you remember, the goal of FBA is to understand the purpose of a respondent's behavior.

Before you can understand the purpose, you must tackle data analysis. Data analysis is the process of synthesizing all the information you have gathered. All of the components that we have mentioned—records, interviews, assessments, and direct observation—are offering you information that point to the function of the student's behavior. But what, exactly, are you looking for?

Once you have compiled this information, you are looking for patterns. You are looking for patterns of your indirect methods of data collection and your direct methods of data collection (Martella et al. 2012). Behavioral patterns are the repeating regularities in acts or actions. Contextual patterns are the repeating regularities of occurrences within the environment. When studying the data you have gathered, you are looking for reoccurrences. Why? Those repeating regularities increase your ability to predict.

Now, we are not fortune tellers, psychics, or magicians. But, the power of a behavioral response pattern to a contextual reoccurrence is prediction. Prediction is what eventually paves the way to understanding the purpose of a target behavior. Today, we are not in need of a crystal ball. We have something far more reliable: data analysis. The success of divining the purpose, so to speak, is the ability to recognize the patterns in the data.

In just a moment, we are going to take you through our method of data analysis. You might have your own way or method. Or, you might work for an organization that mandates you to complete data analysis using their materials. Either way, we are going to take you through the method that has worked for us countless times. Before we delve into these steps, we want to take a moment to warn you that patterns are not always easy to find, and they are sometimes contradictory.

Over the years, we have had those wonderful moments when the contextual-behavioral pattern was obvious. From the first moment of reviewing records, the repeating regularities were practically jumping off the page. Disciplinary forms lined up completely with teacher interviews. When informal assessments were given, the pattern aligned perfectly with the pattern noted in our own observations. The purpose of the target behavior was clear. As the popular saying goes, *"Good times."* When you encounter those moments, smile and enjoy them.

Most of the time, it requires much more work. You have to reflect and critically review the data you have been given multiple times. When this happens, the pattern is more elusive. Other times, there are competing patterns for the same behavior. For example, an interview with a parent and some additional data that have been gathered indicate that a student might use verbal aggression to gain attention. An interview about the same student with a science teacher and some additional data that have been gathered indicate that the student might use verbal aggression to avoid work. In this case, the conflicting information is not wrong. For this student, perhaps verbally aggressive behavior is maintained by both the need to gain attention and the need to avoid work. There are times the same behavior is maintained for different reasons. Remember to use the data to find patterns.

## *Strategy Three: What to Do*

Our system for becoming pattern finders involves four steps: organize data, link data, analyze data, and graph data.

## Organize Data

Are you familiar with the professional organizers who come in and create places in your closet for everything? Before it is over, there are shoe cubbies and drawers for socks. There are different heights of rods that go with pants, shirts, and dresses. There is literally a place for everything! Your closet has been streamlined.

For us, organizing your data is about streamlining the process. You have gained a lot of information, and it has come from a variety of sources. You might have a folder full of random data. In order to streamline the process, each piece of information needs its own place.

We have approached organization by creating a data analysis worksheet. The data analysis worksheet serves three vital functions. First, it allows you to take lengthy interview forms, records notes, and questionnaires and reduce this to a uniformed format. We have found that this allows you to peruse your information in a more efficient manner. Second, the data analysis worksheet allows you to pull out the pertinent information and highlight areas needed for analysis. So, as you read through your indirect sources of data, you simply record your vital information on the form. Third, if you become overwhelmed with the information or cannot remember what information to record, the form guides you through the process. So, you do not have to look back time and time again trying to find the information. You have what you need on the worksheet.

In order to use this form, take out your interviews, records reviews, and questionnaires. If you are working in a team, there is a chance that you were not the person who observed the student or resident. If you were not responsible for the direct observational data, we have provided a place on the form that this can be identified. Then you can use this form as the team analyzes the data. Otherwise, it might be helpful to keep your data separate as you look through your indirect sources of information. So, if you are not using a team approach, only use this form for secondary data sources.

Once you have gathered all of this together, simply go through your gathered information. As you review this data, fill out the form when you come across correlating information. Do not worry; we are not just leaving it at that. We have provided you with the Data Analysis Worksheet in Appendix I. However, in our next section, we will give you a completed form and further explain the worksheet.

If you work in a school or therapeutic environment, your system might already have this tool available to you in a different format. Please use whatever is mandated for your environment. The point of the data analysis worksheet is to keep the process organized and to give you a place to record the pertinent information you receive.

## Link Data

When you were a child, did you ever see one of those holographic images that looked like crazy, squiggly lines with no pattern? Then, some joker told you to put the image to your nose and slowly pull it away. The most amazing thing happened with those squiggly lines. When you slowly pulled the holograph away, an image began to emerge. In the midst of all those squiggly lines, there was a cat, a dog, or a flower! You could not see it at first, but suddenly the pattern was right in front of you!

In data analysis, we are looking to find the patterns or trends in the information we have gathered. Linking is when we begin to see the commonalities emerge. It is that moment of slowly pulling the image away as you begin to have clarity. In order to slowly pull the image away, so to speak, we think you first need to be able to see the complete picture.

Finding the complete picture requires you to see all the information at one time. So, when you complete the data analysis worksheets, you will want to summarize the noted functions for each target behavior. Remember, this is not necessarily your end product. This is not your hypothesis for the target behavior. Rather, this is what you learned from each source. Your secondary sources thought this was the hypothesis for the target behavior.

In order to facilitate this process, we have created a summary sheet to make this step easier. On this sheet, you will write the hypothesized functions of the target behavior for each secondary source of information. This function is derived from the information you have gathered, and researchers have proposed the use of indirect assessment as a way to generate FBA hypotheses (Stage et al. 2002). When you have added the information to the summary sheet, you can quickly see the links or commonalities. You will use data analysis to quantify this information.

Let us give you a quick example. In this hypothetical, you had six sources of secondary information. From five of these sources you derived that the function of the target behavior was maintained by the need to access a tangible item. One source indicated that the target behavior was maintained by the need to gain attention from a teacher. By dividing the respondents who indicated that the target behavior was maintained by the need to access a tangible item by the total number of respondents, you can gain a percentage. Then, you can calculate the total number of respondents who indicated that the target behavior was maintained by teacher attention by the total number of respondents to gain a second percentage. For instance: $5/6 = 0.83 \times 100 = 83\%$, and $1/6 = 0.17 \times 100 = 17\%$. Therefore, 83 % of your indirect sources of information indicated that that the function was to access a tangible item, while 17% indicated it was to gain attention from a teacher.

Remember, you have already reviewed the information from each source, whether quantitative or qualitative. So, when you write down the function from each source, this is not just your opinion. This should be your best estimation applying sound analysis to the process.

As we continue to note, your organization or work setting might have a series of steps and worksheets in place. Even if they do not, you can choose to take your data and complete this step in any way that works for you. Spreadsheets, worksheets, applications, and pencil and paper are just a few of your options. We have created the summary sheet to make this step easier. Linking the information to find the pattern in your secondary sources is your goal. You will find a blank summary sheet in Appendix J. We have provided an example in the application section.

## Descriptive Analysis

We are going to let you in on a little secret; you are technically already analyzing your data. Yep, it is true. That is what you have been doing, but we wanted a place for you to focus on your direct observational data. So, we chose to group it in this section.

As noted previously, observational data are the information that you as the observer or examiner are collecting. It is the descriptive data that are gained from your observations. Descriptive data give the practitioner a means to document the demonstration of challenging, problematic, or interfering behavior and contextual factors (antecedents, consequences) and allow for a measure of magnitude, such as frequency or duration (Steege and Brown-Chidsey 2005). During those observations, you should have completed an antecedent-behavior-consequences (ABC) data collection sheet. Certainly, you might have gathered data on frequency, intensity, and/or duration. However, the ABC model allows the user to record the consequences and actually see the pattern developing. Remember, **A** (antecedent)—**B** (behavior)—**C** (consequence) data collection is about identifying the contextual variables that precede and follow a target behavior. It is a form of data collection requiring the observer to record what happens before the target behavior, during the target behavior, and after the target behavior. Let us go back to Michael talking out. Perhaps the ABC data sheet looks like the one below.

| Antecedent | Behavior | Consequence |
|---|---|---|
| Teacher instructing class on multiplication. | Michael loudly states, "I'm hungry. When are we going to eat." | Teacher verbally redirects Michael to listen. |
| Teacher instructing class on multiplication. She asks a student to work out the problem on the board. | Michael says loudly, "This is boring." | Teacher ignores him. A few students turn and look at him. |
| Teacher asks another student to come to the board. | Michael starts chanting, "Boring, boring, boring!" over and over. | The teacher interrupts Michael and tells him to go sit in the hallway. He does so without hesitation. |

Let us look a little closer at the ABC form. It is clear that math instruction is taking place when Michael calls out.

| Antecedent | Behavior | Consequence |
|---|---|---|
| Teacher instructing class on multiplication. | Michael states, "I'm hungry. When are we going to eat." | Teacher verbally redirects Michael to listen. |
|  |  | *Gains teacher attention* |
| Teacher instructing class on multiplication. She asks a student to work out the problem on the board. | Michael states loudly, "This is boring." | Teacher ignores him. A few students turn and look at him. |
| *Student involvement begins.* |  | *Teacher attention is not gained. Student attention is gained.* |
| Teacher asks another student to come to the board. | Michael starts chanting, very loudly, "Boring, boring, boring!" over and over. | The teacher interrupts Michael and tells him to go sit in the hallway. He does so without hesitation. |
| *Student involvement continues.* | *Intensity and frequency have increased. Escalated behavior. Repetitive and loud chanting with increasing volume.* | *Work avoided; escapes classroom.* |

Let us take a closer look at this scenario. Let us suppose that Michael is seeking attention. The first time he talks out, the teacher verbally redirects him. This is attention. The second time he becomes louder, but he is ignored by the teacher. He does have a few peers who turn to look at him. On the final occasion, he has become escalated and is sent away from everyone. If Michael is trying to gain attention, then the consequence of sending him away from the class to the hall would not maintain his behavior. Additionally, data gathered on different days and at different times will show that he is seeking attention. When attention is given as a consequence, the behavior will continue.

Now, let us suppose that Michael is really attempting to avoid work with his behavior. In the first scenario, the teacher has begun instructing the class. Michael speaks out and is subsequently redirected. As the work becomes more student-involved, Michael actually gets louder. His behavior is ignored by the teacher, but a few peers look at him. As yet another student is called to the board, Michael becomes very boisterous and chants over and over. The teacher sends him to the hallway. In this manner, Michael has successfully avoided his math, including the possibility of working at the board. Now tomorrow, if you were to arrive to observe Michael in math again and the same scenario occurs, a pattern that supports the hypothesis that Michael is talking out and disrupting the classroom to avoid work would begin to form. When work is avoided, the talking out behavior will continue to occur.

As you analyze your data, you are looking for patterns. These patterns will emerge when you can see the consequences that maintain behaviors. In Michael's case, we conclude that the behavior is maintained by consequences that remove Michael from the learning environment. Therefore, his behavior is maintained by the need to avoid work and possibly escape from the classroom.

As part of direct observational data analysis, it is helpful if you do some form of summary so you can have your data in one place (Martella et al. 2012). This helps you to see the commonalities in your information. For this reason, we developed a summary sheet for your direct observational data. This worksheet will be the same as the one for linking indirect sources of information, just designed to address direct observation. Each day of observation, you should be calculating your data. Whether event recording, interval recording, duration recording, latency recording, or ABC data recording, you need to be determining percentages regarding the student or resident's behavior. This information was covered extensively in the previous chapter. If you get lost, pull that information out and read it again. You want to be able to demonstrate in a variety of ways what the student or resident's behavior looks like in the classroom. How pervasive is it? How ongoing is it? What are the percentages for certain antecedents and maintaining consequences? These data are eventually what you will include on your summary sheet and drive the decision-making regarding the target behavior's function. We have included a blank summary sheet in Appendix K. For your informational purposes, we completed one below in the application section.

# Graphing

One of the easiest ways we have found to both look for patterns and demonstrate the data collected in the FBA is to graph. Graphing is the process of using a visual to show relationships. Bar graphs or line graphs are the easiest way to demonstrate multiple data sources side by side. Certainly, you can delve into a variety of graphs with creative color scheming and creative comparison models. However, the goal of graphing is to give you a straightforward picture of the information you have gathered. For the purposes of an FBA, it might be more efficient to use the type of graph you have the most experience in developing. The information is the star; the graph is just the *tool*.

It has been our experience that most organizations dictate this element of an FBA. Many only want line graphs, and even specify what type of program is used in developing the graph. Since this is so pervasive, we advocate for you to follow the specifics suggested by your organization. If for some reason your organization has not determined this, there are so many graphing applications, tools, and resources to choose. Even most word processing programs allow you to insert easy to use graphs. Remember, the visual representation of the data helps you and/or the team to clearly see the pattern emerging in the data. This will be important when you look towards developing a hypothesis statement.

## *Strategy Four: Application*

### Organization

The data analysis worksheet in this chapter organizes information in a very specific manner. For your ease of use, we will advise you on each of the worksheet's components.

*Source* The originator of information. As this book has detailed, there are multiple sources of information: records, informal assessments, interviews with caregivers and staff, and direct observation.

*Target Behavior* The target behavior is the action or act that is interfering with the student's success.

*Characteristics of Target Behavior* We have narrowed this down to five characteristics. Are the behaviors atypical, inappropriate, interfering, uncontrolled, and/or dangerous?

*Absolutes* This is the *always* and the *never*. If there is a person, time, circumstance, and/or situation present *always* and/or *never* when the behavior occurs?

*Setting Events* These are sometimes called distant settings. It is the characteristics—either biological, cultural, medical, or involving a life event—that impact the student and possibly the target behavior.

*Contextual Factors* The person, time, circumstance, and situation in which the target behavior occurs. This is the *who, what, where*, and *when* of the behavior.

*Antecedent* This is what happens before the target behavior. (Since this is not dealing with a specific incident, the antecedent on the summary is what typically happens.)

*Consequence* This is what happens after the target behavior occurs. (Since this is not dealing with a specific incident, the consequence on the summary is what typically happens.)

*To Access, Avoid/Escape, Communicate or Gain/Obtain* On the worksheet, you need to choose one of these.

*Function* What is the student attempting to gain or to avoid?

On the form, you will note that you begin by identifying the source of information and the target behavior that will be addressed on the worksheet. It is important to clearly delineate which behavior is being addressed. Otherwise, data could be lost. The rest of the form offers categories on the areas covered in this book. Simply summarize or note the information received by the source you are recording. Remember, the data sheet is not your hypothesis. Even though you are writing in a function at the end of the form, you are using this to record the information you have received from the sources you used. It is their information, not your information. Below, you will see a completed data worksheet.

**Data Analysis Worksheet**

Source: Type/Position/Name

| Records | Parent/Caregiver | Staff | Direct Observation |
|---|---|---|---|
| IEP | Biological | X    Teacher | Type of Data |
| Disciplinary Report | Foster | ___  Administrator | |
| 504 Plan | Other | ___  Counselor | |
| RTI | Name: | ___  Paraprofessional | |
| Bus Referral | | ___  Other | |
| Medical | Interview/Questionnaire | Name: Mrs. Jones | |
| Attendance | | Interview/Questionnaire | |
| ___ Other | | | |

Target Behavior: Michael talks out loudly and off topic during instruction in all academic areas.

Characteristics: __ atypical  ⬜inappropriate  ⬜ interfering  __ uncontrolled  __ dangerous

Are there times/circumstances/individuals/situations when the target behavior never occurs?

The behavior never occurs in lunch, recess or special areas, such as physical education, music and art.

Are there times/circumstances/individuals/situations when the target behavior always occurs? There are days when the behavior occurs less. But, in all academic areas, Michael will interrupt the teacher more than once daily.

Setting Events:

| Physiological (Medical, Biological) | Cultural (Heritage, Socioeconomic, Religious) |
|---|---|
| None known | Michael does not seem to have any conflicting history that prompts interruptions |
| Pharmacological (Medications, Treatments) | Life Events (Recent Traumatic Event) |
| None known | Parents divorced last year |

Contextual Factors:

| Who (Individuals Present) | What (Events/Occurrence Factors) |
|---|---|
| Teachers, peers | Instruction in all area |
| Anytime an academic areas is addressed | Classroom |
| When (Time of day, Season) | Where (Setting) |

Antecedent:

| Typically academic instruction is occurring | |
|---|---|

Consequence: List the typical responses to the target behavior.

| Teacher/Paraprofessional nonverbal redirection |
|---|
| Teacher/Paraprofessional verbal redirection |
| If Michael persists, then… |
| Teacher stopped instruction |
| Sent away from group/Time out |

Function: Is the behavior to access, avoid/escape, communicate or gain/obtain

| Avoid/Escape | Communicate | Gain/Obtain |
|---|---|---|
| Administrator/School Counselor | Anxiety/Concerns | Administrator/School Counselor |
| Attention | Discomfort | Attention |
| Activity | Dissatisfaction | Activity |
| ☐Academic Task | Physical Pain | Parental Attention |
| Classroom | Response to task, work or request | Peer Attention |
| Discipline | Other: _____ | Place/Setting |
| ☐Instruction | | Situation |
| Parental Attention | | Teacher/Paraprofessional Attention |
| Peer Attention | | Work |
| Place/Setting | | Other: _____ |
| Task | | |
| Teacher/Paraprofessional Attention | | |
| Work | | |
| Other: _____ | | |
| Social Dynamic (Not Attention) | Stimulation | Tangible |
| Power | Repetitive Behavior (flapping, | Activity |
| Control | pacing, rocking) | Game |
| Status | Discontented/Bored | Item |
| Revenge | Impulsive behavior | Money |
| Other: _____ | Other: _____ | Token |
| | | Toy |
| | | Other: _____ |

Function of Behavior: *Michael's behavior is maintained by the need to avoid academic instruction.*

# Linking

Here is the completed summary sheet below. You will see that Michael's records indicated his function was to avoid work. His mom's information pointed to both work avoidance and peer attention. His math and science teacher indicated that his behavior is maintained by the need to avoid work. His reading instructor's information indicated that Michael was attempting to avoid work and gain teacher attention.

**Functional Behavioral Assessment**
**Phase Two: Purpose**
**Data Analysis: Summary Worksheet**

**Name:** Michael Jones                                                    **Date:** March 15, 2016

Target Behavior: Michael talks out loudly and off topic during instruction in all academic areas.

| Source | Avoid/ Escape | Communi-cate | Gain/ Obtain | Social Dynamic (Not Attention) | Stimulation | Tangible |
|---|---|---|---|---|---|---|
| *Records* | Avoid work | | | | | |
| *Parent* | Avoid work | | Gain peer attention | | | |
| *Staff #1 Math* | Avoid work | | | | | |
| *Staff #1 Reading* | Avoid work | | Gain teacher attention | | | |
| *Staff #1 Science* | Avoid work | | | | | |
| *Staff #1* | | | | | | |
| *Staff #1* | | | | | | |
| *Direct Data* | | | | | | |

By using the summary sheet above, we are able to quickly identify that all five sources agree that Michael is attempting to avoid work. Additionally, two sources identify a possible maintaining factor as attention. If you were summarizing 60 % of the indirect sources of information indicated that Michael's target behavior was solely maintained by work avoidance. Additionally, 40 % of the indirect sources indicated that the target behavior was maintained by work avoidance and gaining attention ($3/5 = 0.60 \times 100 = 60\%$; $2/5 = 0.40 \times 100 = 40\%$).

Just one more thought, we have already said it but … this information was derived by reading and analyzing your material. You are using the summary after you have recorded your information, reflected on the information, and summarized the information. This takes time!

**Phase Two: Purpose**
**Data Analysis: Observation Summary Worksheet**

**Name:** Michael Jones                                    **Date:** March 15, 2016

Target Behavior: Michael talks out loudly and off topic during instruction in all academic areas.

| Observation Dates | Avoid/Escape | Commu-nicate | Gain/Obtain | Social Dynamic | Stimulation | Tangible |
|---|---|---|---|---|---|---|
| Observation #1 2/12/16 | Math—Board activity | | | | | |
| Observation #2 2/16/16 | Math—Board activity | | | | | |
| Observation #3 2/17/16 | | | | Gain con-trol—Read-ing group | | |
| Observation #4 2/18/16 | Reading—Group read | | | | | |
| Observation #5 2/19/16 | | | | Science—Teacher attention | | |
| Observation #6 2/23/16 | Math—Inde-pendent work | | | | | |
| Observation #7 2/25/16 | Observed | In | PE | No | Behaviors | Noted |
| Observation #8 2/26/16 | Observed | In | Art | No | Behaviors | Noted |
| Observation #9 3/3/16 | Social stud-ies—Research | | | | | |
| Observation #10 3/7/16 | Math—Inde-pendent work | | | | | |

As part of this method, you should be calculating your ABC chart, frequency, duration, etc., daily. You might not have to use every type of data collection method talked about in Chap. 8, but the ones you do use should be calculated after the evaluation. This is an example, but you should be arriving at your functions based on the calculations you made each day.

For instance, let us use a hypothetical situation. You observed Michael on March 3, 2016. When you reviewed your ABC chart you found that Michael's talking out behavior occurred three times. In all of these instances, it occurred before the teacher asked the class to complete a math problem. Two times the teacher verbally reprimanded him. The last time, Michael was sent to the back of the room and told to put his head down. The next three times the teacher introduced a math problem; Michael had his head down and did not have to participate. He also did not talk out or interrupt. So, three out of six times Michael talked out and interrupted when a math problem was given to the class as an assignment, which is 50% of the time. Two out of three times, the teacher reprimanded him. The final time, Michael escaped from the work by his removal. The teacher did not reprimand Michael again. Michael was not expected to work. Michael did not speak out. When the class was given a verbal directive with Michael expected to participate, 100% of the time he talked out. When the class was given a verbal directive and Michael was not expected to participate, he did not talk out at all, 0%. In the three times Michael was expected to work, the teacher reprimanded him 67% of the time. The last time he was removed from the immediate area of work. During the three times, Michael was not in the immediate area of work, nor expected to work; the teacher never reprimanded him because he never talked out, 0%. Michael was only reprimanded when there was an expectation to work.

## *Strategy Five: What Not to Do*

It is so important to analyze your data with objectivity. The data will point you in a direction. If you have an observation where things do not line up with previous data, do not discard it. It is offering information that is also valuable. If this is the case, ask yourself, *What is different about today? Who is present? What is happening? How are staff and peers responding to the student?* The anomalies can often confirm your data by pointing out the daily differences. These differences could be the impacting factors that need to be changed in order for the student to have success. So, do not skip over anything. Be patient and analyze your information carefully.

## A Before-You-Proceed Checklist

1. Define data analysis.
2. Familiarize yourself with the importance of finding patterns in data analysis.
3. Identify the four steps to finding patterns in data.

**Author Takeaways**
*Takeaway from Stephanie, the behavior specialist:*
   In this chapter, we have provided you with categories for the function of behavior. These are not etched in stone, so to speak. We created these categories to offer a clear and discernible manner in which to conceptualize the function. These can be fluid categories. Use them as organizational tools, not as absolutes.
   *Takeaway from Alan, the school psychologist:*
   It is essential to remember that information may be important, though its importance may not always be evident. You do not want to discount any information simply because it does not seem to "fit." It may be an important piece of the puzzle, though it may not be evident right away. As we said, be patient when analyzing your data.

# References

Johnson, B., & Christensen, L. (2008). *Educational research: Quantitative, qualitative, and mixed approaches*. Thousand Oaks: Sage Publications.

Lichtman, M. (2006). *Qualitative research in education: A user's guide*. Thousand Oaks: Sage Publications.

Martella, R. C., Nelson, J. R., Marchand-Martella, N. E., & O'Reilly, M. (2012). *Comprehensive behavior management: Individualized, classroom, and schoolwide*. Thousand Oaks: Sage Publications.

Stage, S. A., Cheney, D., Walker, B., & LaRocque, M. (2002). A preliminary discriminant and convergent validity study of the teacher functional behavioral assessment checklist. *School Psychology Review, 31*, 71–93.

Steege, M. W., & Brown-Chidsey, R. (2005). Functional behavioral assessment: The cornerstone of effective problem solving. In R. Brown-Chidsey (Ed.), *Assessment for intervention: A problem solving approach* (pp. 131–167). New York: Guilford.

# Chapter 10
# Purpose: Development of Hypotheses

## What You Need to Know

The culmination of functional behavioral assessment (FBA) is the identification of the target behavior's function. In *Purpose,* the practitioner uses data analysis to reach this conclusion. It is at this juncture that we find ourselves.

At the beginning of this book, it was expressed that in its most basic form, FBA can be defined as a multilayered method of determining the function or intent of a behavior. It is a systemized approach that allows the practitioner to answer the question: *What purpose does this behavior serve?* The answer comes in the form of the hypothesis statement.

## Strategy One: Understand the Basics

You might remember from school that a hypothesis is often defined as an educated guess. It is a proposed explanation based on the available data and serves as a starting point for further inquiry. Essentially, you are looking at the evidence you have gathered and drawing a conclusion. As it stands, it is a thoughtful and well-considered conclusion.

## Strategy Two: Understand the Scope

Individuals receiving an FBA often exhibit behaviors that have emerged as challenging within the environment. Whether this is in a school, residential program, home, or the community, these challenging behaviors become roadblocks to the

© Springer International Publishing Switzerland 2016    113
S. M. Hadaway, A. W. Brue, *Practitioner's Guide to Functional Behavioral Assessment,*
Autism and Child Psychopathology Series, DOI 10.1007/978-3-319-23721-3_10

individual's success within the environment (Simonsen and Sugai 2013). The FBA provides important information to move the individual towards greater success within the environment. Specifically, the hypothesis gives those involved with the individual a starting point for building this success. Different members of the team can develop hypotheses, and there is research to support general education teachers' ability to collect data and generate hypotheses after receiving training (Maag and Larson 2004; Moore et al. 2002; Packenham et al. 2004).

The development of a reliable hypothesis statement is the next step in behavior planning. This book has guided you in the FBA process. If the information from the FBA was not channeled to help with programming and curriculum, it would be at best an information-gathering mission; at worst, packed away and never considered again. FBA is not an intervention or single strategy (Nelson et al. 1999); rather, it is a process. So, it is important to think of the FBA as part of a broader spectrum of tools leading to a goal. We have named the steps to lead you through our ideology. Here they are again.

**Process** ⇨ **Purpose** ⇨ **Planning** ⇨ **Prevention**

It has been established that the hypothesis statement identifies the Purpose of a student's behavior. This information is formed from careful analysis of the information gathered regarding an individual's behavior. Once the purpose has been defined in the form of a hypothesis statement, the team can use this information to predict the instances, people, situations, and settings that maintain the behavior (Ryan et al. 2003). Once these contextual factors are understood, the team can then plan on the measures that will be put in place. These measures could include interventions, strategies, curriculum, modifications, and accommodations, which serve to prevent behaviors that will disrupt the success of the student.

## Strategy Three: What to Do

For the purposes of FBA, the hypothesis statement takes all the information that has been painstakingly analyzed and summarizes it succinctly. Effective hypotheses concisely identify the main thrust of the target behavior. This summary statement emerges from analysis, but do not forget that it is a hypothesis; it is the considerate and thoughtful "best guess" resulting from analysis. A three-step process is outlined by the hypothesis statement: When *something* occurs, the student does *something*, in order to achieve *something*.

## *Characteristics of an Effective Hypothesis*

*Accurate* It is important that the hypothesis statement emerges from three areas: accurate data, accurate analysis, and an accurate statement. If you are concerned about accuracy in any of these areas, it is important to revisit them. It is far better to take time to complete additional observations or further data analysis than to overlook the errors and provide an inaccurate reason for the target behavior. Inaccurate information on every level, including the hypothesis statement, will impact the planning phase of behavioral programming. At some point, all efforts will prove ineffective and the target behavior could actually become more frequent or intense due to inaccuracy.

*Clear* The hypothesis statement should address the target behavior. Be certain to clarify which target behavior is being addressed. The hypothesis statement is also identifying the contextual factors involved in maintaining the target behavior. If there are contextual factors that are pertinent in maintaining a behavior, make certain that the hypothesis statement is clear on these factors.

*Concise* The hypothesis statement should be concise. You have gathered quite a bit of information, but too much information tends to overcomplicate the hypothesis statement. This makes it difficult for others to use the statement effectively.

*Easy to Understand* The hypothesis statement should be understandable for every user. You might have the ability to develop a deep, thoughtful statement that would rival any academic. However, if it is not understood by the people who are responsible for implementing behavior plans, it will be irrelevant. Keep these things in mind when developing your statement.

In an earlier chapter, we introduced a function chart for guidance as part of a worksheet. When writing a hypothesis statement, this chart can help you identify the function of the target behavior. We have included it in Appendix L. We offer it here for guidance.

First, ask yourself: *Is the behavior to avoid/escape, communicate, gain/obtain, or access?*

Second, choose from the list. If the function is not on the chart, write in your own.

| Avoid/Escape | Communicate | Gain/Obtain |
|---|---|---|
| Administrator/School Counselor<br>Attention<br>Activity<br>Academic Task<br>Classroom<br>Discipline<br>Instruction<br>Parental Attention<br>Peer Attention<br>Place/Setting<br>Task<br>Teacher/Paraprofessional Attention<br>Work<br>Other: _____ | Anxiety/Concerns<br>Discomfort<br>Dissatisfaction<br>Physical Pain<br>Response to task, work or request<br>Other: _____ | Administrator/School Counselor<br>Attention<br>Activity<br>Parental Attention<br>Peer Attention<br>Place/Setting<br>Situation<br>Teacher/Paraprofessional Attention<br>Work<br>Other: _____ |
| Social Dynamic (Not Attention) | Stimulation | Tangible |
| Power<br>Control<br>Status<br>Revenge<br>Other: _____ | Repetitive Behavior (flapping,<br>pacing, rocking)<br>Discontented/Bored<br>Impulsive behavior<br>Other: _____ | Activity<br>Game<br>Item<br>Money<br>Token<br>Toy<br>Other: _____ |

As you know, there are contextual factors, setting events, and other types of information that you might want to add to the FBA. You can do this in the form of background information; or if there is contextual information that needs to go along with the hypothesis, you can give a clearer definition in a summary statement after the hypothesis. That way any clarifying details you need to add can be included near the hypothesis statement. We will include this in Approach C in the Application portion of the chapter.

## Strategy Four: Application

We have seen hypothesis statements written in many different ways. Each way has its advantages and disadvantages. For this chapter, we have chosen to outline a step-by-step process for you. Certainly, there are many ways to approach this. If you have a form from your state or district, use what is mandated or required. Below you will see four different ways to approach the development of the hypothesis statement.

### *Approach A*

Scenario: Carol pushes other students when lining up for a transition. After analysis, it has been determined that Carol is attempting to be closer to the teacher.

Step one: Identify if the target behavior is occurring to avoid/escape, communicate, gain/obtain, or access something.

Result: *Carol pushes other students when lining up to gain....*

Step two: Identify the goal of the behavior. What is the individual attempting to avoid/escape, communicate, gain/obtain, or access? In this area, the possibilities are endless. Use your analysis to make your determination. Below you will find a list of the more common reasons:

| Avoid/Escape | Communicate | Gain/Obtain |
|---|---|---|
| Administrator/School Counselor<br>Attention<br>Activity<br>Academic Task<br>Classroom<br>Discipline<br>Instruction<br>Parental Attention<br>Peer Attention<br>Place/Setting<br>Task<br>Teacher/Paraprofessional Attention<br>Work<br>Other: _____ | Anxiety/Concerns<br>Discomfort<br>Dissatisfaction<br>Physical Pain<br>Response to task, work or request<br>Other: _____ | Administrator/School Counselor<br>Attention<br>Activity<br>Parental Attention<br>Peer Attention<br>Place/Setting<br>Situation<br>Teacher/Paraprofessional Attention<br>Work<br>Other: _____ |
| Social Dynamic (Not Attention) | Stimulation | Tangible |
| Power<br>Control<br>Status<br>Revenge<br>Other: _____ | Repetitive Behavior (flapping, pacing, rocking)<br>Discontented/Bored<br>Impulsive behavior<br>Other: _____ | Activity<br>Game<br>Item<br>Money<br>Token<br>Toy<br>Other: _____ |

After analysis, it has been determined that Carol is attempting to be closer to the teacher. She is attempting to gain teacher attention.

*Hypothesis statement: Carol pushes other students when lining up to gain teacher attention.*

## *Approach B*

Step one: List the target behavior.

Step two: List the hypothesis statement following the above example.

Step three: List the response.

*Result:*

*Target behavior: Carol uses her hands to push other students when directed to line up for a transition throughout her school day.*

*Hypothesis statement: Carol's behavior is maintained by her need to gain attention from her teacher.*

*Response: When Carol gains attention from her teacher, she quits pushing other students.*

## *Approach C*

_____ (Insert student name)'s _____ (behavior) is maintained by her need to

_____ (avoid/escape, communicate, gain/obtain or access) _____ (insert:

attention, work, place, item, person, communication need, tangible or social dynamic word).

*Result:*

*Hypothesis statement: Carol's pushing behavior is maintained by her need to gain attention from her teacher.*

What if the target behavior serves more than one function?

If the target behavior serves more than one function, add this to the hypothesis statement.

Scenario: Carol pushes other students when lining up for a transition. She also pushes them when they have a toy. After analysis, it has been determined that Carol is attempting to be closer to the teacher. She is also attempting to take the toy and play with it.

*Result:*

*Hypothesis statement:*

*Carol's pushing behavior is maintained by her need to gain attention from her teacher and access a toy.*

*Summary: Carol's pushing behavior primarily centers on gaining teacher attention. During direct observation, 67 % of the target behavior was in conjunction with moving closer to the teacher. Even though there was not a lot of time in her school day to play, it was noted that she pushed other children 56 % of the time during recess. Out of this 56 % of the time, Carol was always attempting to gain access to a toy. She used her pushing behavior to force other children to give her the item in their hands. In all cases, this was a toy. She did not exhibit any preference for a specific toy. She just seemed to want to gain access to the toy. In this manner, Carol's pushing behavior serves both the function to gain teacher attention and access a toy, typically from another student.*

## Strategy Five: What Not to Do

1. Be unclear
2. Be too wordy
3. Be inaccurate
4. Base the hypothesis on opinion alone

## A Before-You-Proceed Checklist

1. Understand what a hypothesis statement is.
2. Be able to use the function chart provided in the chapter.
3. Be able to write a hypothesis statement.

**Author Takeaways**

*Takeaway from Stephanie, the behavior specialist:*

The hypothesis statement is the launching point of behavior planning. Take your time when developing it. It needs to be balanced giving a brief, concise, and accurate understanding of the target behavior to those who will use it. Remember, though, it is a hypothesis. If new data and behavior disprove the hypothesis, that is okay. This is not a rigid, one-time-only statement. It is fluid, as is behavior. Behavior changes. If the target behavior evolves, there is no harm in revisiting the hypothesis statement. As a student matures and contextual factors change, the hypothesis statement might change as well. It is better to revise and make the process fluid than remain rigid about findings… especially those that are identified as a hypothesis anyway.

*Takeaway from Alan, the school psychologist:*

Sometimes hypotheses are correct, but sometimes they are incorrect. As you gather additional data, your working hypothesis may change and evolve into something else. It may actually go in a completely different direction. This is fine. Go where the data are, because when you do, you are likely to be able to make better sense of what you know about the student, even if it is not what you originally thought.

## References

Maag, J. W., & Larson, P. J. (2004). Training a general education teacher to apply functional assessment. *Education and Treatment of Children, 27,* 26–36.

Moore, J. W., Edwards, R. P., Sterling-Turner, H. E., Riley, J., DuBard, M., & McGeorge, A. (2002). Teacher acquisition of functional analysis methodology. *Journal of Applied Behavior Analysis, 35*(1), 73–77.

Nelson, J. R., Roberts, M. L., Mathur, S. R., & Rutherford, R. B. (1999). Has public policy exceeded our knowledge base? A review of the functional behavioral assessment literature. *Behavioral Disorders, 24,* 169–179.

Packenham, M., Shute, R., & Reid, R. (2004). A truncated functional behavioral assessment procedure for children with disruptive classroom behaviors. *Education and Treatment of Children, 27,* 9–25.

Ryan, A. L., Halsey, H. N., & Matthews, W. J. (2003). Using functional assessment to promote desirable student behavior in schools. *TEACHING Exceptional Children, 35*(5), 8–15.

Simonsen, B., & Sugai, G. (2013). PBIS in alternative education settings: Positive support for youth with high-risk behavior. *Education and Treatment of Children, 36*(3), 3–14.

# Part IV
# Phase III: Planning

**Professional Responsibilities** Within *Planning*, the practitioner would lead the team in the review of the functional behavioral assessment and developing interventions based on the hypothesis statement.

**Alternative View** The *Planning* phase could also be considered the *implementation phase*. This phase is about leading, reviewing, developing, and planning.

**Task List**
1. Gather Team
2. Complete FBA
3. Review FBA
4. Write BIP

**Goal** By the end of this phase, the practitioner will have gathered and led the team in developing a behavior intervention plan.

---

*Planning* is the third phase and a step just beyond writing a functional behavioral assessment.

# Chapter 11
# Planning: Deconstructed Functional Behavioral Assessment

In this chapter, we are going to break down the components of a sample functional behavioral assessment (FBA) for Jason Peterson. This example should give you a better idea of the complexity of an FBA as well as help you to understand the information that should go in each section.

## Part 1: Assessment Procedures

In this section, you will list the components of your FBA.
   Example:

**Assessment Procedures**
School record review
Parent, student, and teacher interviews
Functional Analysis Screening Tool (FAST)
Collection and analysis of anecdotal record
Direct behavior observation

## Part 2: Referral Information

In this section, you will discuss the reasons why an FBA was requested. You should address the student's current educational services, describe the behaviors, and provide as many details as possible.
   Example:

**Referral Information**
Jason is a 6-year-old male in kindergarten at Meadow Elementary School. He was referred for an FBA by his classroom teacher, Mrs. Nancy Miller. Mrs. Miller reports that his challenging behaviors have been present since August 2015. The

© Springer International Publishing Switzerland 2016                                    123
S. M. Hadaway, A. W. Brue, *Practitioner's Guide to Functional Behavioral Assessment,*
Autism and Child Psychopathology Series, DOI 10.1007/978-3-319-23721-3_11

referral information received identifies Jason's target behaviors as (1) crawling on the floor—under the classroom tables, (2) making animal noises that distract class and instruction, and (3) shouting out—interrupting. In February 2016, Jason became eligible for exceptional education services through the Other Health Impairment program.

## Background Information

### Physical

Jason's mother reports that he does not have any current health-related illnesses. His vision and hearing are reportedly adequate. Jason has been given diagnoses of attention-deficit/hyperactivity disorder (ADHD) and oppositional defiant disorder. In the past, he has taken medication to address his behavior. His mother reports that it has been difficult to find a medication that effectively treats Jason's symptoms.

### Academic

Presently, Jason participates in a kindergarten classroom at Meadow Elementary School. He did attend prekindergarten (Pre-K) through the district's Pre-K program. This year, Jason has struggled to attend to his academic tasks. His frequent off-task behaviors appear to have led to academic difficulties. In the area of reading, Jason began the year identifying 40 letters; his goal was 50. When tested mid-year, Jason had only gained 3 points with a score of 43. In the area of initial sound fluency, Jason had identified 15 words with a goal of 26 by the end of the year. As of his last evaluation, he has not made any progress and remains at 15 words. Jason has improved his sight word recognition and timed random letter recognition. He has improved from 4 sight words to 10 and from 2 recognized letters to 17 this year. In the area of math, testing indicates that Jason has been inconsistent in his progress. When tested on random number recognition, Jason went from 8 out of 20 recognized to 7 out of 20 recognized.

### Behavioral

Both Jason's mother and teacher report that he exhibits disruptive and active behavior at home, at school, and in the community. He "talks constantly" and will frequently interrupt classroom instruction. Jason also makes animal noises and shouts out in class. If he does not want to participate in an activity, he might yell out, "I don't want to!" He often modifies assignments, locations, and tasks to his preferences. Frequently, he refuses to comply with the first request from an adult. During these times, he might verbally refuse or negotiate for a different assignment.

Additionally, Jason is described as being in "constant motion." He will crawl under tables and scoot across the room in his chair. Jason will often run from his teacher in the hallway. If an adult attempts to retrieve him, Jason will grab hold of items refusing to return with the adult or remain with his class. At home, Jason exhibits many of these same behaviors; however, his mother reports that he has more leisure time and places to move around, such as his trampoline. She does report that his behavior escalates in the community. Often, he will make noises and attempt to engage strangers in public places. It is further noted that his behavior can become aggressive. When escalated, Jason might hit others with his bookbag or squeeze another student's hand or arm tightly. Jason also has difficulty following directions and waiting for his turn in an activity.

# Part 3: Operational Definition of Target Behaviors

In this section, you will define the target behaviors. An operational definition is important to help clarify the problematic behaviors that the student is displaying. Be as detailed as possible when you discuss these behaviors; this information will be very important to you as you work through the remaining sections of the FBA.

Example:

**Operational Definitions of Target Behaviors**

In an effort to adequately address Jason's behavioral needs, the target behaviors received in the referral packet have been reviewed. The original behaviors reported have been adapted, combined, and operationalized to provide a more comprehensive functional assessment. The new target behaviors along with their operationalized definitions are reported below.

**Target Behavior One: crawling on the floor—under the classroom tables**

- Jason crawls, walks, skips, and runs away from his directed or assigned area both inside the classroom and outside of the classroom. This also occurs during instructional, academic, and transitional times.

**Target Behavior Two: making animal noises**

- Jason makes animal noises and other types of sounds both inside the classroom and outside of the classroom. This also occurs during instructional, academic, and transitional times.

**Target Behavior Three: shouting out—interrupting**

- Jason calls out right and/or wrong answers without permission, talks off topic, shouts, screams, and verbally interrupts adults and students inside the classroom and outside of the classroom. This also occurs during instructional, academic, and transitional times.

# Part 4: Previous Intervention Strategies and Consequences

In this section, you will discuss the intervention strategies and consequences that have been used in the classroom. Be sure to list things that were and were not effective. In addition, you will describe any terms that would likely be unfamiliar to teachers and/or parents.

Example:

**Previous Intervention Strategies and Consequences**
Interviews with both Mrs. Peterson and the school staff indicate that numerous intervention strategies have been attempted with Jason. Mrs. Peterson reports that Jason has been under a doctor's care and treated with medications. She further reports that the medications have not consistently improved Jason's overall behavioral challenges. She reports, "His body seems to metabolize the medications too quickly." Within the home, Jason's behavior has also been addressed through corporal punishment, grounding, positive rewards, ignoring less aggressive behaviors, and restrictions. Although discipline continues to occur, it does little to reduce the frequency of Jason's behaviors. Mrs. Peterson reports that his behaviors are a constant at home. At school, Jason's teacher reports the same. Mrs. Miller identifies constant movement and talking as significant challenges within the learning environment. To address these and other concerns, Jason participates in a check-in–check-out plan with the school counselor. He also has access to a behavior chart and a token economy reward system. In addition to this, Jason receives verbal warnings and redirections when his target behavior is evidenced. Other strategies the school system has used include, but are not limited to, the following: verbal praise and redirection, office referrals, calling Jason's parents, suspension from the school bus, classroom rules, and school-wide rules. As with the home interventions, the wide range of behavioral strategies used at school have done little to improve Jason's behavior.

# Part 5: Assessment Summary

In this section, you will provide a summary of the data you collected as part of your assessment. Interviews, questionnaires, and observations will be included here. Since this section has the most information, it will be the largest part of your FBA.

Example:

**Assessment Summary**
*Anecdotal Methods*
Jason's mother, teacher, and Jason were all interviewed either through questionnaire, over the phone, or in person about their concerns and perceptions regarding Jason's behavior. All adults noted positive traits about Jason. He is described as a friendly student with a lot of potential. Jason's behavior has presented challenges for him in the home, the school, and the community. Both his mother and teacher

report that he appears to be seeking attention. When in the community and at school, Jason often attempts to gain the focus of others. His mother reports that he becomes increasingly anxious and/or fidgety in public. At times, he will walk up to complete strangers and begin to make noises. This noise-making behavior is replicated within the school environment. At school, Jason has become aggressive by hitting others with his bookbag, pushing, and squeezing other students. He is disruptive and will attempt to escape from his teacher. Jason also has difficulty waiting for his turn. Both at home and school, he demonstrates a preference for "having things his way." He can become oppositional when this is challenged.

As part of the FBA process, Jason was also interviewed. He was very responsive to the interview process. Jason reports that he likes to ride his bike, jump on the trampoline, and play. His favorite thing at school is "playing in the gym." Jason easily differentiated between appropriate and inappropriate behaviors. He reports that he was on "green" the day of the interview. Prior to that time, "I was on red three days." To him, red means, "You don't do good. Then, your mom or your dad gives you a whooping!" He reports that he, "Don't do what I was supposed to do." Jason further states that his misbehavior happens because, "I do it so I can be laughing." He goes on to say that only one student laughs with him. When asked about how his teacher feels about his behavior, he states, "She is happy." As for his mother, "She feels happy too." As for himself, "I feel happy." When given three wishes, Jason reports that he would like, "A horsie, a Shetland pony. I want worms, lures. I want baseballs. I have a bat, but I lost my baseballs. I want to have a kid table, one of those that are circled. Oh, I wish for a guitar too."

As part of the interviews, Jason's teacher, mother, and counselor were all given assessments and a rating scale to complete based on the target behaviors identified earlier in this report. The rating scales were given in an attempt to isolate the function of Jason's behavior during school. The information gathered from the returned scales is reported below.

*The FAST* is an assessment tool that identifies environmental and physical factors that may influence problem behaviors. Participants are asked to identify the problem behavior including frequency, intensity, situations, antecedents, and consequences. They are then asked to answer 16 Yes/No questions. These answers are placed into categories of Attention/Preferred Items, Escape, Sensory Stimulation, and Pain Attenuation. The answers are then used to identify potential sources for the function of the problem behavior.

It is noted that all three respondents ranked Attention/Preferred Items as the highest ranking. One respondent ranked Escape as equal to Attention. In addition to identifying possible functions for target behavior, the *FAST* allows respondents to identify other behavior descriptors. At school, Jason's behaviors can occur throughout the day and in different areas of the school. His behaviors are seen as "mild" with disruption but little risk to property and health to "moderate" with property damage or minor injury. Disruptive behaviors could include yelling out, making noises, and crawling under the tables. Out of all three respondents, no one identified Pain Attenuation as a possibility for the function of Jason's behavior (Fig. 11.1).

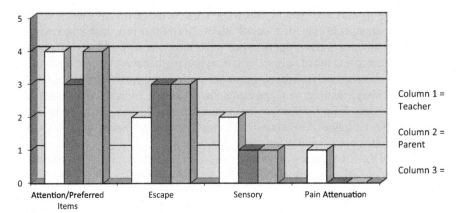

**Fig. 11.1** The Functional Analysis Screening Tool

**Descriptive Analysis**

Jason was observed on seven separate occasions over the period of 3 weeks. These observations took place at various times throughout Jason's school day. He was observed in his classroom, transitioning in the hallway, and during physical education. On all occasions, Jason demonstrated all of the identified target behaviors.

The Target One behaviors deal specifically with Jason leaving his assigned area. They have been operationalized as, "Jason crawls, walks, skips, and runs away from his directed or assigned area both inside the classroom and outside of the classroom. This also occurs during instructional, academic, and transitional times." Throughout the observational period, Jason was typically moving in some form. Data were not gathered on all movement. For instance, if Jason asked permission to get an item or object and skipped across the room, these data were not collected. Rather, movement that involved Jason leaving his area without permission was the focus of this targeted behavior. During seven observational periods, Jason exhibited the targeted behavior a total of 56 times. Each separate observation period lasted between 30 min and 1.5 h.

It is noted that although the behavior was reduced with kinesthetic activities in the classroom, it was not eliminated. Even when given the opportunity to move, dance, or make hand motions during an activity, Jason continued to exhibit some of the Target One behaviors. Also, Jason's most frequent occurrence of this behavior occurred during physical education. When given the opportunity to crawl on the mat, often Jason would roll across the floor. The presence of movement combined with a more unstructured activity increased Jason's Target One behaviors. By the end of the class period, Jason was not maintaining his personal space and became more aggressive when putting his hands or feet on other students.

The Target Two behaviors are identified as making animal noises. They have been operationalized as "Jason makes animal noises and other types of sounds both inside the classroom and outside of the classroom; and during instructional, academic, and transitional times." During all seven observations, these behaviors were observed. More specifically, Jason exhibited a total of 73 behaviors that involved making sounds or animal noises. This occurred irrespective of environmental factors, such as setting, peers, or instructor present.

In conjunction with the Target Two behaviors, the Target Three behaviors also deal with verbal output. They have been operationalized as, "Jason calls out right and/or wrong answers without permission, talks off topic, shouts, screams, and verbally interrupts adults and students inside the classroom and outside of the classroom; and during instructional, academic, and transitional times." During the observational period, Jason exhibited a total of 145 incidents of the Target Three behaviors. The highest incident of these behaviors occurred during whole-group time or whole-group instruction. Jason demonstrated these behaviors with and without redirections from the teacher. During one instructional period, Jason had 52 incidents of verbal output. Within this context, 32 of these behaviors were attempts to directly engage the teacher or a peer. There were 15 episodes of animal noises or sounds. The remaining 7 verbal episodes did not involve any other person. Jason simply talked out loud.

# Part 6: Hypothesis

In this section, you will discuss your hypotheses for why the student is acting in a particular manner. Use your knowledge of behavior and information you collected in the assessment to create your hypotheses statements.

Example:

**Hypothesis**
**Target Behavior One: crawling on the floor—under the classroom tables**

- Jason crawls, walks, skips, and runs away from his directed or assigned area both inside the classroom and outside of the classroom. This occurs during instructional, academic, and transitional times.
  **Target Behavior Two: making animal noises**
- Jason makes animal noises and other types of sounds both inside the classroom and outside of the classroom. This occurs during instructional, academic, and transitional times.
  **Target Behavior Three: shouting out—interrupting**
- Jason calls out right and/or wrong answers without permission, talks off topic, shouts, screams, and verbally interrupts adults and students inside the classroom and outside of the classroom. This occurs during instructional, academic, and transitional times.

**Hypothesis Statement** Jason's behavior is maintained by the need to gain or access attention, to gain or access an item of preference or a preferred encounter, and/or difficulties in inhibiting his impulses.

Primarily, the function of Jason's Target One, Target Two, and Target Three behaviors is maintained by his difficulty in inhibiting his impulses. As noted on the physician form and as part of the eligibility, Jason has been identified as having symptoms associated with ADHD. Often, individuals with ADHD experience problems with executive functioning. Within the context of Jason's behavior, his symptomology cannot be fully separated from his behavioral function. There is, at least in part, behavior that is directly or indirectly impacted by ADHD. This condition appears to shape Jason's interactions at home, at school, and in the community. Therefore, understanding the function of Jason's behavior should begin with a certain weight or consideration being given to symptoms emerging from ADHD, specifically the difficulty of inhibiting his impulses.

Additionally, Jason's behavior is also maintained by the need to gain attention, an item of preference, or a preferred encounter. According to data collected, Jason's persistence to task is limited. He has difficulty attending for prolonged periods of time. This is further complicated by his need to gain attention, an item of preference or a preferred encounter, or even experience. In many instances, this desired encounter is a level of engagement with his teacher. During one of Jason's more disruptive days, 62% of his behaviors were an attempt to gain teacher attention. Therefore, when Jason is presented with a work task, his competing predisposition and preferences limit his interest and ability to stay involved in a lesson or task. The function of Jason's targeted behaviors is to continue to access a preferred internal experience, encounter, or event. He wants to engage the teacher or other students because it is stimulating and satisfying to him. He wants to crawl under tables because he enjoys the experience. It has been noted that behavioral interventions have been largely unsuccessful with Jason. These plans are reported to only work for a limited amount of time. Given Jason's limited persistence to task, it seems that Jason's preferences then outweigh the cost or reward of previous strategies.

Along this line, Jason's behaviors seem to escalate the longer he is denied access to a preferred item, encounter, or experience. Ignoring his behavior does not typically reduce his behavior. His difficulty with impulse control appears to impact him significantly. During his interview, Jason continually talked about play in relation to school and home. Although he demonstrated a conceptual understanding of the purpose of school, his preferences to play and to the types of activities he enjoys dominated his conversation. Just acknowledging the purpose of school does not preclude a student to school appropriate behavior. Rather, Jason's school behavior is dominated by his need to gain attention and high preference encounters. This is also seen in the community. Jason's mother reports that he becomes increasingly fidgety within the community. He will often attempt to gain attention from strangers by deliberately making noises. When someone new comes to their home, Jason will also demonstrate the same type of behaviors. This indicates that he is overstimulated by new encounters, desires attention, and has difficulty inhibiting his impulses.

# Part 7: Recommendation

In this section, you will discuss your recommendations, which will be based on all available data you have collected as well as parts 1–6 of your FBA.

Example:

**Recommendations**

In regard to Jason's unique needs, consider creating a culture of prevention for him. It has been established that he has a history of behavior that has presented challenges within the learning environment. In regard to the function of Jason's behavior, it seems that they are maintained by the need to gain or access attention, to gain or access an item of preference or a preferred encounter, and/or difficulties in inhibiting his impulses. Within Jason's classroom, he would benefit from several environmental elements that will promote prevention. Although his behaviors stem from several sources, developing an effective plan will incorporate his needs for daily, predictable routines. Visual representations, pictures, cue cards, and boundaries will help Jason remember the rules and expectations in his work environment. He would benefit from a visual that would always indicate the expectations and pattern of his day.

Additionally, Jason needs to increase his ability to self-regulate. Presently, he is responding to his environment while ineffectively coping with his difficulty inhibiting his impulses. His processing deficits impact his ability to transition from assignment to assignment, from whole-group to individual work, and from his classroom to other areas of the building. Jason would benefit from three different types of strategies. One strategy would be the manner in which instruction is delivered. Jason needs to be given both verbal and visual instruction. His attention needs to be secured and directions should be simple and clear. He will not be able to successfully move from one instructional lesson to an activity unless this takes places. Second, Jason needs previewing strategies for transition and work. He needs to be cued prior to his turn or a transition occurring. This could take the form of saying, "Jason, get ready. I am coming to you next." Finally, Jason would benefit from skill development. Consider implementing a social skills opportunity for Jason. Groups or supportive materials which promote insight into body awareness and self-regulation would seem appropriate for Jason. Social stories and modeling may also become important avenues to help him. He also demonstrates a need to learn how to develop appropriate and sustainable friendships. Overall, continue to promote positive activities with positive peer interactions, clear social rules, and boundaries for Jason.

Due to Jason's need to gain attention and access to preferred experiences, consider implementing a scheduled "attention" routine. This could take the form of verbal praise or other types of attention that are routinely implemented. Since it is important for Jason to develop socially within his learning environment, another dimension that meets his functional needs is to create social experiences for him. This could take place with some type of supervised play, perhaps playing a game with Jason and one other student. This will help to create opportunities to work on concepts such as sharing or waiting his turn.

It has been noted that Jason is an active student. However, his behavior does not improve with unstructured movement. It might improve with structured movement. If appropriate, Jason's team might want to consider requesting an occupational therapy consult. With or without a consult, Jason seems appropriate for items or experiences that help him cope with his own needs. Consider a wiggle seat, an exercise time, or access to other types of items to improve these concerns. Also, consider giving Jason movement breaks. To encourage self-regulation and self-advocacy, consider incorporating opportunities for spontaneous requests. For instance, Jason would benefit from access to break cards to initiate a request.

Although Jason has not responded successfully to behavioral strategies, he still would benefit from some type of reward or level system. He does not attribute much value to any of the school activities aside from the opportunity of play. By developing an appropriate reward/token system for Jason, there is a related value that is added to his school behavior. By consistently working a plan based on his preferences, he might begin to attach more value to self-regulation and school appropriate behavior.

At one time, Jason was receiving support from a medical doctor for his ADHD symptoms. If at any time he begins receiving services again, it would be helpful for this information to be shared with Jason's school team.

In summary, all individuals associated with this FBA have commented on how much potential Jason does exhibit. It has been a pleasure to interview Jason and everyone associated with this FBA.

# Chapter 12
# Planning: Willow Wilding Case Review (FBA and BIP)

In this chapter, we are going to complete our case study on Willow Wilding. In Appendix M, you can find the functional behavioral assessment (FBA) form used in this chapter. In Appendix N, you can find the behavioral intervention plan (BIP) form used in this chapter.

Here is the culmination of your work with Willow Wilding. We took the liberty of giving you a name. So, Chris Ohno, this is what you worked tirelessly on over the last many weeks.

### Functional Behavioral Assessment
Process, Purpose, Planning, Prevention

**Student Name:** Willow Wilding    **DOB:** 06/01/2008    **Date:** October 1, 2015

Participants present (name and title)

Drew Wilding—Father
Michelle Wilding—Mother
Priscilla Huffing—General education teacher
Donny Data—Behavior interventionist
Latonya Hayes—Occupational therapist (OT)
Gwen Gillespie—Lead special teacher
Chris Ohno—Special education teacher
James Jackson—Speech language pathologist

## Process (List Target Behavior(s) Along with Operationalized Definitions.)

*Target One Behavior* Destructive behavior—Willow uses her hands and feet to turn over furniture, such as desks and chairs, tear items off the wall, and rip up items, such as schoolwork, books, and papers throughout her school day. Baseline data

© Springer International Publishing Switzerland 2016
S. M. Hadaway, A. W. Brue, *Practitioner's Guide to Functional Behavioral Assessment,*
Autism and Child Psychopathology Series, DOI 10.1007/978-3-319-23721-3_12

indicate that Willow's behavior occurs on average 42% of her school day. Further analysis indicates that although the behavior occurs throughout her school day, the majority of the behavior occurs after 12:00 p.m.

*Target Two Behavior* Out-of-area behavior—Willow leaves her assigned area without permission throughout her school day. Baseline data indicate that Willow's behavior occurs on average 63% of her school day. Further analysis indicates that although the behavior occurs throughout her school day, the majority of the behavior occurs after 12:00 p.m.

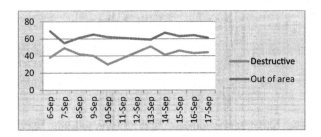

## Data Collection

### *Indirect Assessment*

**Record Review Summary: Circle All That Apply**
Information attained from the following records—medical, assessment, Individualized Education Program (IEP), disciplinary reports

Willow is a seven-year-old female in the second grade at Good Hope Elementary School. She is currently in Mrs. Huffing's classroom. She has been receiving services through the Significant Developmentally Delayed program since first grade. Willow also receives an hour of speech language services and an hour of occupational therapy support weekly. Presently, Willow is supported for two segments of co-teaching in an inclusive environment.

When Willow was tested to determine her eligibility for exceptional education services, her scores indicated that she had average intelligence. Her primary difficulties were in attention to task, social adjustment, and behavioral functioning.

Willow has perfect attendance for both kindergarten and first grade. She has not been absent this school year. She had attended school in a neighboring county until midway through her first grade year. At both her previous school and Good Hope Elementary, Willow has a history of disciplinary reports for both destructive and disruptive behavior. She was suspended 2 days last school year. The first incident was for throwing items and accidentally hitting another student. The second was for running from the school building into the road when she was angry at her teacher. Other than these two instances, Willow has not hurt another student. She has never run from the school building again.

Willow appears to be in excellent health, and there are not any outstanding medical issues at this time. She does not appear to have any limitations in the area of hearing or vision. She is not taking any medications.

**Interview Review Summary: Circle All That Apply**
Information attained from Drew and Michelle Wilding, Priscilla Huffing, and Willow Wilding

As part of the FBA process, Willow, her teacher, and her parents were all interviewed about her behavior. Mr. and Mrs. Wilding and Mrs. Huffing all reported positive things about Willow. She has a fun personality and is often quick to help other students. She likes to play and is often creative. She is a good artist and is on grade level in all areas. She loves to play board games and always responds well to extra computer time. Willow has one sibling, a baby brother who is 2 years of age. She loves spending time with him.

Mr. and Mrs. Wilding report that Willow exhibits many of the same difficulties at home that she does at school. She is often careless with household items and has broken many objects within the home. She cannot be allowed to play outside because she will leave the yard. One time, Mrs. Wilding received a phone call while Willow was playing outside. When she returned, Willow was four houses down the road talking with a group of older children. It took Mrs. Wilding about 20 min to force Willow to return home.

At school, Willow will leave her assigned area without permission. She will run and skip around the room and tear items off the wall. She is loud at times and has broken several objects, including a school-issued electronic tablet. Mrs. Huffing reports that daily Willow tears up items and turns over furniture.

At home, Willow has a set bedtime and chores. However, she exhibits difficulty in these areas. Willow struggles to follow a routine and will not complete her chores without constant encouragement. At school, Mrs. Huffing has also noticed that Willow will not finish her class work without constant redirection. At times, Willow will respond to positive praise and receiving rewards. But, her attention to task is limited and she will quickly lose track again. At both home and school, Willow has been disciplined through receiving consequences. She has lost computer time at home and computer time at school. This seems to only minimally work.

Willow was also interviewed about her behavior. She reports that she enjoys school and that she has a lot of friends. Her favorite part of school is recess. She does not like it when she gets in trouble and has to go to see the principal. Willow reports that she does have problems at school. She understands that she gets out of her seat. She explains, "I just get so tired of sitting. I get all itchy. Like I just want to jump up and down." She does think that her teacher is, "Mad at me. She talks loud to me. Like she doesn't like me." Willow states, "I think that is because I mess up her stuff. But, I just get so itchy. After a long time of being good, I just can't help it. I don't want to do more school work! It gets boring." When asked about what her teachers think about her behavior, Willow states, "They wish I would just sit down." When asked what other students think about her behavior, Willow says, "They start getting mad at me. But, I can't help it!" Willow says that her favorite toys are dolls, board games, and the computer. She also likes when other people say nice things to her.

**Assessment Summary: Circle All That Apply**
Name(s) of assessment: Functional Analysis Screening Tool (FAST)
    Mr. and Mrs. Wilding, Mrs. Ohno, and Mrs. Huffing were all given the FAST.
    *The FAST is an assessment tool that identifies environmental and physical factors that may influence problem behaviors. Participants are asked to identify the problem behavior, including frequency, intensity, situations, antecedents, and consequences. Then, the participants are asked to answer 16 Yes/No questions. These answers are placed into categories of attention/preferred items, escape, sensory stimulation, and pain attenuation. The answers are then used to identify potential sources for the function of the problem behaviors.*
    Target One Behavior

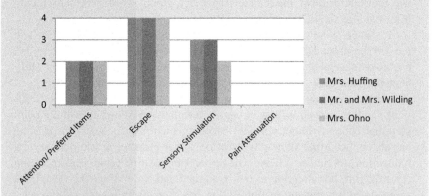

Within the *FAST,* all individuals ranked escape as the most likely function of Willow's behavior. Additionally, Mrs. Huffing and Mr. and Mrs. Wilding ranked sensory stimulation as the second most likely function. Mrs. Ohno ranked attention/preferred items and sensory stimulation as the same. It is noteworthy than no one felt that pain attenuation could be the cause of Willow's behavior.

Target Two Behavior

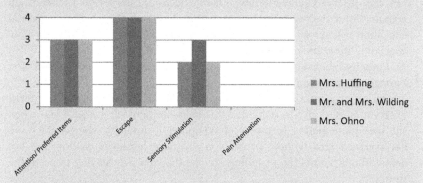

Within the *FAST,* all individuals ranked escape as the most likely function of Willow's behavior. Attention/preferred items were ranked second. Mr. and Mrs. Wilding also ranked sensory stimulation the same as attention/preferred items. Again, no one felt that pain attenuation could be the cause of Willow's behavior.

In addition to identifying possible functions for target behavior, the FAST allows respondents to identify other behavior descriptors. At school, Willow's behaviors can occur throughout the day and in different areas of the school. Her target one behaviors can include property damage and/or minor injury when she allows herself to lose control.

## Direct Observation

**Observation Summary: Gwen Gillespie, Lead Special Education Teacher**
Willow was observed ten times over a period of 3 weeks. During the ten times of observations, either or both the target one or target two behaviors were noted. Willow was observed across settings and in various academic and nonacademic tasks. She was observed in independent work, group work, whole-group instruction, and transitioning. She was observed in the hallway, the classroom, recess, and in computer technology. During the time of observation, there was a teacher and sometimes two teachers present.

Target one behavior: Willow uses her hands and feet to turn over furniture, such as desks and chairs, tear items off the wall, and rip up items, such as schoolwork, books, and papers throughout her school day.

During observation, Willow's target one behaviors were noted on six out of ten observations. She did not exhibit this behavior at recess, computer technology, and on two days of classroom instruction. On both of these days, Willow was observed in the morning. On one occasion, she was in a small group activity within the regular education setting. This group was led by the special education teacher with two other peers present. On the second day, Willow was doing independent work.

Target two behavior: Willow leaves her assigned area without permission throughout her school day.

During observation, Willow's target two behaviors were noted for every observation period. She exhibited this behavior across settings. Even when she was participating in recess or computer technology, she would leave her assigned area without permission. In these instances, Willow left her area without permission or telling anyone that she was leaving to go to the restroom.

Additional observations:

Willow often appeared to grow increasingly restless near the end of the school day. This appeared to be noticeably different than her peers. She typically responded well to verbal praise but did not respond well when corrected. She also did not respond well when given multiple redirections to return to work. Willow was often eager to help and seemed to be very friendly. She loved extra attention but this did not guarantee that she would remain on task. Willow seems to do very well drawing. A follow-up talk with the art teacher found that Willow excels in this area. (Further analysis in the next section.)

## Purpose

**Data Analysis**

Target one behavior:

Antecedent–behavior–consequences (ABC) data were collected on Willow's behavior. On all occasions, Willows behavior was preceded by at least two requests to return to her work. The consequences ranged from moving her color to verbal redirection. Willow did not demonstrate any target one behavior unless this antecedent was in place. Hundred percent of the time, Willow's behavior followed two or more work requests. All of these behaviors occurred after 12:00 p.m.

Target two behavior:

ABC data were collected on Willow's behavior. As for the antecedents, 70% of her behaviors were preceded with a work directive or a teacher request. Twenty-seven percent seemed to occur when other children were getting teacher attention. The last 3 % occurred when Willow wanted to sharpen her pencil, go to the restroom, or get something without asking permission. Consequences typically entailed verbal redirection, verbal reminders, or changing her color, depending on the severity of Willow's behavior

Target one behavior: Willow uses her hands and feet to turn over furniture, such as desks and chairs, tear items off the wall, and rip up items, such as schoolwork, books, and papers throughout her school day.

Hypothesis statement: Willow's behavior is maintained by her need to avoid a work request or task directive and a non-preferred situation.

Explanatory summary: The function of Willow's target one behavior is avoidance. On almost all occasions since the beginning of the school year, Willow has responded destructively to two or more directives or redirects. Additionally, she has exhibited these at-risk behaviors primarily in the afternoon. According to Willow's OT, she further seems to experience more fatigue than other students. The more fatigued she becomes, the more likely she will be to react to non-preferred tasks with a higher number of redirects. Given her low endurance for attention to task, Willow's behaviors seem to be compounded later in the day.

Target two behavior: Willow leaves her assigned area without permission throughout her school day.

Hypothesis statement: Willow's behavior is maintained by her need to avoid a work request or task directive and a non-preferred situation.

Explanatory summary: The function of Willow's target two behaviors is avoidance. Just as her target one behaviors are to avoid tasks, requests, or non-preferred situation, so are her target two behaviors. Willow seems to exhibit these behaviors with more frequency than the target one behaviors. The behaviors occur throughout the day, while the majority of the target one behaviors occur in the afternoon. This seems to be because fatigue increases the severity of the avoidance behaviors. Also, even though this is not the primary reason, Willow has exhibited a need for attention when the target two behaviors are exhibited.

## Planning

Target one behavior: Willow uses her hands and feet to turn over furniture, such as desks and chairs, tear items off the wall, and rip up items, such as schoolwork, books, and papers throughout her school day.

> Brief summary of recommendations: Willow needs a consistent reinforcement plan to address behaviors. Although a token economy has been attempted, the team feels that Willow might benefit from a punch card system that allows her to earn a mark or punch on the card for demonstrating correct behavior. She also needs to begin to understand her own triggers and feelings of fatigue.

Target two behavior: Willow leaves her assigned area without permission throughout her school day.

> Brief summary of recommendations: Willow needs a consistent reinforcement plan to address behaviors. Although a token economy has been attempted, the team feels that Willow might benefit from a punch card system that allows her to earn a mark or punch on the card for demonstrating correct behavior. She needs to be given breaks throughout her school day.

## Prevention (Changes Made to the Environment's Climate, Culture, and Community.)

Target one behavior: Willow uses her hands and feet to turn over furniture, such as desks and chairs, tear items off the wall, and rip up items, such as schoolwork, books, and papers throughout her school day.

> Prevention plan: Willow needs a skill-training segment. Consult with the OT for ideas to help with her fatigue and attention to task. Consider some form of self-mediation to address the intensity and destructiveness Willow exhibits. Develop a safety plan along with Willow to aid in this regard.

Target two behavior: Willow leaves her assigned area without permission throughout her school day.

Prevention plan: Willow needs a skill-training segment. Consider working with Willow on understanding her need to move. Work on developing activities and learning opportunities that are more enjoyable for Willow. Complete a personal preference inventory to gain an idea of her likes and dislikes.

*Meeting date for BIP:* October 14, 2015

Other: (concerns, comments, looking ahead statements)
   Over the next 2 weeks, the ideas suggested will be implemented to determine if these should be used on the BIP. Consider implementing an opportunity to draw and create as part of her plan

As it turns out, the team did meet on October 14, 2015. Here is the BIP that you led them to create. By the way, the next chapter is going to help you in the development of a BIP. Consider this a precursor with Willow. Again, you will find a blank copy of this form in Appendix N.

**Functional Behavioral Assessment**
**Phase Three: Planning**
**Behavior Intervention Plan**

**Student Name:** Willow Wilding     **DOB:** 06/01/2008     **Date:** October 14, 2015

Participants present (name and title)

Drew Wilding—Father
Michelle Wilding—Mother
Priscilla Huffing—General education teacher
Donny Data—Behavior interventionist
Latonya Hayes—OT
Gwen Gillespie—Lead special teacher
Chris Ohno—Special education teacher
James Jackson—Speech language pathologist

Target one behavior: Destructive behavior—Willow uses her hands and feet to turn over furniture, such as desks and chairs, tear items off the wall, and rip up items, such as schoolwork, books, and papers throughout her school day. Baseline data indicate that Willow's behavior occurs on average 42% of her school day. Further analysis indicates that although the behavior occurs throughout her school day, the majority of the behavior occurs after 12:00 p.m.

Function of behavior: Willow's behavior is maintained by her need to avoid a work request or task directive and a non-preferred situation.

Antecedent modifications (list all that apply): Social skills to include triggers and self-mediation, fidget to address OT recommendations, chill-out spot to give her a place for a break, visual schedule with special highlights to indicate when she will receive a break, and school work that involves more kinesthetic activities.

Replacement behaviors:

Willow will keep her hands and feet to herself.

Willow will request a break when she needs one (to be taught with social skills).

Willow will respect her property and the property of others by handling it with care.

Reinforcers: punch card system—Willow will earn a punch on her "You can do this!" card when she (1) uses an appropriate behavior, such as request to take a break, (2) goes 30 min without a target one behavior. When a line is filled, Willow chooses from a motivator list that includes: computer time, board game with a friend, extra break time, and free motivator choice.

Consequences: When an infraction occurs, Willow will receive a redelivery of a social skill related to the infraction. Willow will not earn a punch on her "You can do this!" card. Depending on severity, her parents will be notified.

Target two behavior: Willow leaves her assigned area without permission throughout her school day.

Function of behavior: Willow's behavior is maintained by her need to avoid a work request or task directive and a non-preferred situation.

Antecedent modifications (list all that apply): social skills to include requesting permission and self-mediation, fidget to address OT recommendations, chill-out spot to give her a place for a break, visual schedule with special highlights to indicate when she will receive a break, and school work that involves more kinesthetic activities

Replacement behaviors:.

Willow will raise her hand to ask permission to leave her assigned area. Willow will request a break when she needs one (to be taught with social skills).

Reinforcers: punch card system—Willow will earn a punch on her "You can do this!" card when she (1) uses an appropriate behavior, such as request to take a break, (2) goes 30 min without a target one behavior. When a line is filled, Willow chooses from a motivator list that includes: free time for artwork, computer time, board game with a friend, extra break time, and free motivator choice.

Consequences: When an infraction occurs, Willow will receive a redelivery of a social skill related to the infraction. Willow will not earn a punch on her "You can do this!" card. Depending on severity, her parents will be notified.

Plan of action (method of data collection, personnel involved, progress monitoring parameters, reporting): Frequency data will be collected by all of Willow's teachers. This will be collected and monitored at the end of every week by Willow's case manager. All teachers will use the "You can do it!" card throughout Willow's day.

Parents will receive a daily report card identifying Willow's progress with the "You can do it!" card. Data on the overall plan will be reported when progress notes are sent home by the school. On this form, progress will be reported in the progress monitoring section.

Target one: Baseline data indicate that Willow's behavior occurs 42 % of her school day.

Goal: When the data indicate that there is a 50 % improvement, the team will revisit this plan.

Target two: Baseline data indicate that Willow's behavior occurs 63 % of her school day.

Goal: When the data indicate that there is a 40 % improvement, the team will revisit this plan.

---

Progress Monitoring:

Date: _____ Progress: _____

Date: _____ Progress: _____

Date: _____ Progress: _____

Date: _____ Progress: _____

Additional Information: _____

_____

_____

# Chapter 13
# Planning: Writing a Behavior Intervention Plan

## What You Need to Know

Designing effective behavioral strategies is a critical extension of the functional behavioral assessment (FBA) process. An FBA gives the practitioner important information on the contextual factors regarding the target behavior. Without this information, the behavior intervention strategies will be ineffective (O'Neill et al. 2015). The hypothesis statement presents a theory as to the contextual factors that prompt and sustain the target behavior. Understanding the situations, people, and events that sustain the target behavior allows the team to predict when these behaviors will most likely occur. Once this prediction is made, the team is set to develop effective planning to lessen or resolve the target behavior.

## Strategy One: Understand the Basics

Behavior planning varies greatly from state to state and from district to district. Along with this variability come legal mandates and district requirements that differ significantly. Additionally, environmental factors such as an educational setting, a residential setting, or a treatment setting might also dictate the types of strategies and interventions that are appropriate, required, and accessible to a team (Simonsen and Sugai 2013). What will work in one setting might not work in another. What is feasible in one location might not be in another. So, before beginning the task of behavior planning, it is important that you determine the requirements and guidelines in your area. There might be helpful forms available to you within your own organization. Or, your district might leave much of this up to your or a support team's discretion. Whichever is the case, knowing this will set you up for success in the planning stages.

For our purposes here, we will consider behavior planning as the process of creating and/or modifying an individualized program designed to address the target behaviors identified in the FBA. Within the parameters of behavior planning,

© Springer International Publishing Switzerland 2016
S. M. Hadaway, A. W. Brue, *Practitioner's Guide to Functional Behavioral Assessment,*
Autism and Child Psychopathology Series, DOI 10.1007/978-3-319-23721-3_13

we believe that the successful practitioner will address four areas: the individual, baseline data, the environment, and programming. Much of this information will have been gleaned from the FBA process. So, there is no need to reinvent the wheel. Thorough interviews and record searches will have given you a lot of this information. Just in case this might seem unclear, we recommend that your planning include the following:

**Individual** Functional assessments have shown progress in improving behavior in children (Blair et al. 1999). However, this is not a generalized process; you are focusing on the individual. You are looking for influencing factors such as medical conditions, medications, treatments, traumatic events, or life changes. Additionally, you would want to consider cognitive functioning, learning difficulties, and skill acquisition. Specifically, what academic, social, and emotional skills does the individual possess or still need to develop?

There are two types of deficits that are commonly discussed among Individualized Education Program (IEP) and support teams: a skill deficit and a performance deficit. A skill deficit exists when a student or resident does not know how to perform the behavior or task that is being requested or expected of them. Generally, a skill deficit stems from insufficient opportunities or appropriate avenues to learn the skill (Gresham and Elliott 1989). A performance deficit exists when a student or resident does know how to perform the behavior or task that is being requested or expected of them but chooses not to do so. It is imperative that the team understands which deficit the student is exhibiting. Each requires a different strategy and approach.

**Baseline Data** The starting point for developing a plan is to have the original baseline data from the FBA. The baseline data is the rate or measure of the target behavior prior to the implementation of any type of intervention (Cipani and Schock 2010). It is impossible to evaluate a plan's effectiveness unless you know how often the target behavior occurred.

**Environment** You are looking for contextual factors. When these conditions are in place, the individual exhibits the target behaviors. These predictive conditions are the *who, what, when*, and *where* of the environment. You are focusing on time of day, setting, personnel involved, and the activity that is taking place.

**Programming** You are considering rewards and consequences, curriculum to teach skills, changes in placement, modifications to the environment, accommodations within the environment, strategies, developing a behavior intervention plan (BIP) and how to teach the student replacement behaviors.

With all of these components, it is important to understand that this is not just a review of knowledge; the team is considering how to design these elements for prevention. First, how will the team teach the individual replacement behavior, skill development, and self-management? Second, how will the team create an environment that supports prevention for the individual?

## Strategy Two: Understand the Scope

Certainly, behavior planning can be a timely process. In most environments, supports have been developed to address and streamline the process. Within the school system, behavior planning can be integrated into the IEP. Students with disabilities who have become eligible for a special education program will have an IEP in place. Within the IEP, behavior planning can be addressed through accommodations, modifications, personnel training and supports, a BIP, transportation, and goals. Even for individuals without an identified disability, understanding and designing programming might be beneficial. Although it might not be legally mandated, as is the case with an IEP, this type of investment is certainly an investment worth undertaking.

There are many strategies that can be implemented to address the occurrence of a target behavior. Newcomer and Lewis (2004) found that interventions are more effective when they are created to address the function of target behaviors than those that do not address the function of target behaviors. Skill teaching, goal setting, and reinforcers are all excellent strategies to help reduce and possibly eliminate target behaviors. Many of these strategies can be outlined in the form of a BIP. The BIP is a tool that details all the specifics of a behavior plan for a student exhibiting problematic behaviors. The BIP specifically identifies the target behaviors and gives a detailed description of how the target behaviors will be managed in the environment. The BIP governs the response of all staff members when the individual exhibits the target behavior. This provides much-needed consistency and uniformity. Without consistency and uniformity, negative behavior is reinforced. When a BIP is part of a student's programming with an IEP, it becomes a legal requirement for the student's team. It is not just something that is put down on paper; it is the mandate for how the target behavior will be handled.

## Strategy Three: What to Do

There are as many different formats and ways to write BIPs as you can imagine. Some suggestions include the following steps: review the targeted behavior, determine behavioral goals, identify intervention strategies and personnel responsible for implementation, identify dates to review the plan, and determine methods for evaluation of the plan (Fad et al. 1998). Within the school system, the Individuals with Disabilities Education Improvement Act of 2004 (IDEA 2004) does not give a specific format requirement for a BIP. Because of this, there is frequent variability from state to state, as has been mentioned. Your state or district might require you to use a specific form or format; these are typically designed to make the process easier. We have included a sample BIP form in Appendix N. In contemplating the BIP, it seems to us that there are certain areas that should be addressed. If these are addressed, no matter what format you choose, then the plan should contain everything that is needed.

**Step One** Identify the individual. Be sure to place the name or identifying case number of the student on the BIP.

**Step Two** Indicate the date. It will be helpful to indicate the date that the plan was put into place.

**Step Three** Identify the target behavior(s). Simply state the measurable and concrete definition that was used as part of the FBA process. If there was more than one, list them as Target Behavior One, Target Behavior Two, and Target Behavior Three. It is generally accepted that no more than three target behaviors should be listed on the BIP. The team could decide to add more, but it is very difficult to work on more than three behaviors effectively.

**Step Four** Identify the function of the target behavior(s). This is your hypothesis statement. (Do you see how you can just plug the FBA information into the BIP?)

**Step Five** Identify modifications to the antecedent. Let us go back for just a minute. Do you remember what an antecedent is? It is what happens right before the target behavior occurs. It is *where* the student is, *who* is around, *what* activity is taking place, and *when* all of this is happening. We have used a few different terms for the antecedents. One of them is contextual factors. Contextual factors could include objects, people, events, tasks, directions, time of day, behavior of other people, physical location, and many, many more factors.

When an FBA is in process, a significant portion of the analysis should reveal these contextual factors. When writing a BIP, this information is reviewed and considered. Research has indicated that manipulating the antecedents is useful in BIPs (Conroy and Stichter 2003). Therefore, the team should modify the contextual factors to aid in the prevention of the target behavior. These might range significantly depending on the target behavior. However, here is a list of a few to give you a clearer example: altering physical location, completing a preferred preference inventory, introducing a sensory-related item, creating a cool down or safe spot, teaching social skills, altering the length of an assignment, using previewing strategies, creating a visual schedule, training in calming techniques, using break cards, giving the student choices, and many, many more. It will be up to the team who is developing the BIP to determine the most appropriate modifications to be implemented.

**Step Six** Identify replacement behavior(s). All target behaviors serve a purpose. As it has been detailed, that purpose is to *avoid/escape, communicate, gain/obtain*, or *access*. Since the need that prompts the target behavior might not be eliminated, it is important to teach the individual alternative behaviors to replace the faulty target behaviors. For example, Lauren is a sixth grade student. She wants the teacher to work with her on division. So, every time a math lesson begins, she yells out for help. An acceptable alternative behavior would be for Lauren to raise her hand when she needs help. She still needs help, but raising her hand is a more appropriate means to gain help.

Replacement behaviors are the alternative behaviors that are preferable in the learning environment (Gresham et al. 2001). They are behaviors that need to be taught and then positively reinforced. When considering the development of the alternative behaviors, the team needs to make certain that the replacement behaviors can be taught and are accessible in the environment. The team also needs to ensure that these behaviors are true replacement behaviors and will serve the same function as the target behavior(s). Additionally, the team needs to define specifically what the replacement behaviors are and develop a plan to teach or encourage the use of these behaviors. A few examples of acceptable, alternative behaviors are as follows: raising hand, keeping hands and feet to self during transition, asking to go to a cool down spot, using a break card, using respectful language, writing in a journal, requesting time in the sensory lab, requesting to speak with the school counselor, and many, many more.

**Step Seven** Identify reinforcers and a reinforcement schedule. A reinforcer is a consequence that increases the likelihood of a behavior. During the development of a BIP, the team has already decided interventions through the modification of the antecedent and the identification of replacement behaviors. In order to increase the likelihood that the replacement behaviors will occur, the team will need to consider the types of reinforcements appropriate for the intervention plan.

There are several ways to approach reinforcements, but as is the case in all intervention planning, the reinforcers need to be accessible and appropriate for the environment in which they will be used. When introducing reinforcement, it needs to be delivered immediately and consistently (Jolivette et al. 2000). Also, the team needs to consider the preferences of the individual. When preparing for this type of planning, the team could consider using a personal preference inventory. This inventory will be a brief survey that indicates what the student enjoys most. For instance, does the student value attention over a tangible item? Does the student like working on the computer more than playing a game with a friend? Understanding the preferences of the individual will help the team determine effective reinforcers.

Next, the team should determine a reinforcement schedule. There is no doubt that you have already heard of a reinforcement schedule. It has been our experience that people often get concerned about their ability to understand how to choose a reinforcement schedule. To break this down, let us begin with a good definition for a reinforcement schedule. At its most basic, a reinforcement schedule defines when an individual will receive the reinforcer. It determines how often this exchange will occur. As you might suspect, it can become a little more complicated. Do not be concerned! The team needs to determine what will be most effective.

**Continuous Reinforcement** A continuous reinforcement schedule is when a replacement behavior is reinforced every time it is exhibited. For instance, Lauren wants help in math class so she yells out. The team determines that Lauren's replacement behavior should be raising her hand. When Lauren raises her hand to gain help, the teacher verbally praises her and gives her the help she needs. The teacher administers this reinforcement every time Lauren raises her hand for help in math. Therefore, there is continuous reinforcement when the replacement behavior is demonstrated.

Since the replacement behavior is reinforced every time it is exhibited, a continuous reinforcement schedule is often effective when teaching a new behavior and teaching a young student. Since the reinforcement is given only in relation to the desired behavior, the student most likely will begin to make an association between the new behavior and the reinforcement. Although this is advantageous during reinforcement, it does not usually create lasting change. The strength of the schedule is in helping the student to link the replacement behavior with a preferred reinforcer.

**Ratio Reinforcement** A ratio reinforcement schedule is when a behavior is reinforced after a specific number of occurrences. There are two types of ratio reinforcement schedules: fixed ratio and variable ratio. A fixed-ratio reinforcement schedule is when the reinforcer is given after a fixed number of occurrences. It could be the second, third, or fifth time the replacement behavior occurs. This is up to the discretion of the behavior team. The important thing is that the reinforcer is delivered systematically. Going back to Lauren in the math class, every third time Lauren raises her hand in class, the teacher would give her verbal praise. She would not get verbal praise on the second time or seventh time. Only on every third occasion that Lauren raises her hand. The obvious advantage of this type of reinforcement is that it helps to establish a contingency between the replacement behavior and the reinforcer. It is critical that the reinforcer is delivered consistently. Otherwise, this will prove unsuccessful in behavior change. Additionally, a fixed-ratio schedule is really a step in behavior planning. The goal is to increase the likelihood of the replacement behavior without a reinforcer. Therefore, the fixed-ratio schedule is not a lasting solution and should not be used over extended periods of time.

The second type of ratio reinforcement schedule is the variable reinforcement schedule. This schedule is similar to the fixed ratio, but the reinforcer is only applied after the replacement behavior is exhibited an approximate number of times. In Lauren's case, she is receiving the reinforcer three times. She is stepped down to a variable-ratio reinforcement schedule, so she is receiving the reinforcer approximately every three times. So, Lauren might receive the verbal praise on the fourth time she raises her hand and then on the sixth time. It still occurs, but not with the rigid frequency as before. Since the reinforcer is not given on a consistent basis, this schedule would be somewhat ineffective in teaching a new behavior. It would make the contingency between the replacement behavior and the reinforcer less pronounced. This schedule is beneficial when fading out a more rigid schedule, such as the fixed-ratio reinforcement schedule. It allows the user to identify the progress the student has made in generalizing a behavior.

**Interval Reinforcement** An interval reinforcement schedule is when a replacement behavior is reinforced after a period of time. It is appropriate for any behavior that involves duration, such as working on task for a specified time. There are two types of interval reinforcement schedules: fixed interval and variable interval. A fixed-interval reinforcement schedule is when the reinforcer is given after the replacement behavior has been demonstrated for a predetermined period of time. For instance, Ahmed is restless and gets out of his seat frequently during a test. When Ahmed sits in his seat for 10 min without getting up, he is given a sticker as a reinforcer. The amount of time is determined based on baseline data that has been gathered and the discretion of the behavior team. Just as with a fixed-ratio reinforcement schedule, the important thing is that the reinforcer is delivered systemati-cally. The advantage of this type of reinforcement is that it helps to solidify a newly emerging replacement behavior. Since the behavior is often contingent on the rein-forcer, the replacement behavior might stop if the reinforcer is stopped. Therefore, the fixed-interval schedule is not a lasting solution. Once the replacement behavior has increased, consider moving towards a variable-interval reinforcement schedule.

As with the fixed-interval reinforcement, there are similarities between the vari-able-interval reinforcement and variable-ratio reinforcement. A variable-interval re-inforcement is given after an average length of time, not a specified length of time. Ahmed might receive the sticker after 8 or 11 min. Since the reinforcer is not given after a specified amount of time, consider the appropriateness when working on a new behavior that requires duration as a key to success. It is quite appropriate to use the variable-interval reinforcement schedule when a student is ready to move into a less rigid schedule of reinforcement. If a student is unsuccessful as the reinforce-ment is faded, they have not generalized the replacement behaviors.

Before leaving this topic, please remember that all reinforcers and reinforcement schedules need to be accessible in the environment. If the schedule or reinforcer is unrealistic, it will not be used with consistency. Consistency is the key to success. Inconsistency will reinforce the behavior that you do not want to emerge.

**Step Eight** Identify the consequences. Consequences are sometimes a tricky technique that can lead to a very slippery slope. Research has indicated that some school-based personnel choose punitive and exclusionary measures regardless of the identified function of a target behavior (Scott et al. 2005). After countless meet-ings to discuss behavioral strategies with school teams, it has been our experience that people gravitate towards more restrictive consequences. Therefore, it is impor-tant to differentiate between a consequence and a punishment. They are not the same. They are not words that can be exchanged with the same meaning.

| Consequences | Punishment |
| --- | --- |
| Teaches | Dictates |
| Allows the student an element of control | All control is given to the punisher |
| Based on rational or logical sequences | Based on the will of the punisher |
| Focuses on positive language | Often uses reactive language |
| Teaches natural order | Demands compliance |
| Chooses thinking over feeling | Chooses feelings and emotional responses, such as anger |

Consequences are not always negative; there are many consequences that are posi-tive. Every day we are the recipients of consequences based on our own actions. They happen so often that we do not usually think about them. If we pay the power bill, our electricity stays on. If we go to work, we get paid at the end of the month. Consequences follow a logical sequence. For example, if Gerard arrives late for school, he must go to the office for a tardy slip. This is a natural consequence of arriving late.

With the development of a BIP, consequences are preferable over punishment. They are preferable because they teach rather than just enforce. Punishment has an aversive quality. It is often based on pain or discomfort. This pain or discomfort is used as a deterrent to the unwanted behavior. If a student is the recipient of a punishment, it might stop the behavior in the moment. However, it does not necessarily offer lasting change. The aversive does not offer the "teachable" moment. It does not instruct the student on how to do better. Rather, it enforces compliance through discomfort or pain.

When the team considers consequences for the occurrence of the target behavior, think of strategies rather than payback. Think of natural and logical rather than rigid and unbending. For example, when an infraction or target behavior occurs, an acceptable consequence would be to have a social skill delivered that matches the infraction. When it was Dion's turn, Joanie yelled out the answer before he could respond. So, on Joanie's turn, Dion gets to answer. Since Joanie is a repeat offender and is working on interrupting and yelling out, she will receive a mini-lesson on interrupting behavior.

Consequences need to be:

1. *Communicated clearly to the student*—The student needs to be educated on the consequences that will be a part of his/her behavior intervention. Part of the teaching element necessitates that the student has accountability for his own behavior. Unless the student understands that when the target behavior occurs the identified consequence will follow, the consequence might become just another form of random punishment.

2. *Related to the infraction in a logical manner*—When a consequence relates closely to the target behavior, two things happen. It is easier to understand the link between the two, and the "teachable" moment is more understandable. Unrelated consequences are hard for the student to understand and might come across as retaliation and punishment.

3. *Accessible in the environment*—Here is the bottom line on accessibility: If a consequence is not appropriate, attainable, or available in the environment, then it cannot be used effectively. If a consequence cannot be used effectively, then it cannot be systematically applied. If a consequence is not systematically applied, it will increase negative behavior. Therefore, every consequence should be appropriate, attainable, and available in the environment.

4. *Systematically applied*—When you teach any skill—behavioral or academic—a key to success is consistency. In the case of behavior intervention, the consequence is applied in response to the target behavior. When the target behavior occurs, the consequence should be executed as stated in the BIP. Without the systematic application of the consequence, the consequence will be ineffective. For example, Ronaldo changes classes four times a day. If the intervention plan states that Ronaldo's consequence is that he does not earn a token when he refuses to line up for class change, every teacher has to execute this same consequence when Ronaldo does not line up for class. Otherwise, the consequence will not be effective.

5. *Contain an instructional element*—Teachable, teachable, teachable! The strength of using a successful consequence rests in the opportunity to instruct the individual regarding decision-making, problem-solving, and the impact of the target behavior on the individual, others, and the environment. If the consequence is only about taking something away or adding something aversive when a target behavior is exhibited, then that begins to seem a lot like punishment. The consequence is a tool to teach behavioral change. Finding the teachable moment is key when choosing consequences for the BIP.

6. Never used as a form of retaliation—Just in case it has not been clear, punishment and consequences are not interchangeable words or actions. A consequence is not given to "get back at" or "show the student who is boss." Acceptable consequences will be free of retaliatory motives. Otherwise, a power struggle will ensue. In a power struggle, each party is attempting to "win" the battle. This approach destroys effectiveness and breaks apart trust.

**Step Nine** Plan of Action. The final step in the development of the BIP is the plan of action. A BIP is fluid. One should not be written and remain without evaluation. If the plan is not working, the target behavior resolves or a new target behavior emerges, the BIP should be reassessed and changed based on need. The plan of action is what guarantees that these eventualities are monitored. It outlines the methods by which the BIP will be monitored and evaluated.

First, the plan of action details the manner in which data will be collected. It identifies how the data will be collected, who will collect the data, and who will review the data. For data collection, the team might use a variety of means including, but not limited to these few: behavior monitoring forms (behavior charts, points sheets, tally marks, punch cards, etc.), student self-assessment and/or progress monitoring forms, observations, attendance records, and disciplinary records. This information needs to be monitored by one person. In most instances, there is a case manager, teacher, counselor, or other type of point person who will take the lead. This person is responsible for collecting the data and reviewing the data. If the BIP involves an individual who goes from place to place, it is likely that each class or training environment will have someone who gathers data on the BIP. This person might be a teacher who uses a behavior-monitoring sheet for the period the student is in her class. Then, the point person will gather and review the information from every class or training environment as the plan dictates. When reviewing this information, the team lead is looking for progress, lack of progress, and the emergence of new behavior. It is impossible to know if progress has been made unless you first know the baseline data. Be sure to have this information available each time data is reviewed. Without it, the team lead will be uncertain of progress. Also, the schedule for gathering the data from each person responsible varies based on student need. It could be that the plan is reviewed by the team lead daily, weekly, or monthly. It is our preference that the data are gathered from all sources and reviewed by the point person at least weekly. A great deal can happen and change in a month. Monitoring the plan closely increases awareness and insight into its effectiveness.

Second, the plan of action details how the team will handle the information reviewed by the team lead. This involves how progress will be communicated to all interested parties, including parents and caregivers. This also involves identifying any type of evaluative measures that might be implemented to monitor progress. The team might also consider how long it takes before the plan is changed based on lack of progress. Be careful, though—it takes a while for a plan to be effective, and progress can be slow. It is important that the team gives it a chance to work.

**Step Ten**  Include the names of everyone involved in the development of the BIP. Often, the BIP will be developed as part of an IEP meeting. So, there should be a signature sheet available. We have seen both a signature sheet and a BIP with a place for every name on the actual BIP. Bottom line: include the names of everyone involved in the development of the BIP.

Although technically not listed on a BIP, durability is a necessary component to success. As we noted, it is important for the consequences to be consistent. However, it is important for the dutiful execution of the plan to continue over a period of time until no longer needed. Research has indicated that longevity is important to a BIP's success (Kern et al. 2006).

## Strategy Four: Application

If you are in the school system, chances are that your district has provided a BIP form that simply needs to be filled out. We have seen dozens of these forms, and they vary significantly in requirements and formatting. Do not let the format throw you off! Generally, the forms require about the same type of information. Just in case, we have provided a few versions that we created for your review.

**Target Behavior**  Kevin pushes and kicks with his hands and feet other students during free play, including in the classroom and on the playground and throughout the school day when free play is given.

**Function of Behavior**  Kevin's behavior is maintained by the need to gain access to a tangible item (usually a toy).

**Antecedent Modifications**  (List all that apply.)
Social skills training
Modeling to address sharing and accepting "no" from a peer.
Prior to free play, Kevin will choose three toys that will stay with the teacher for free play. Kevin will have the opportunity to ask the teacher for one of the toys. Then, trade it for another if he chooses throughout free play.
Kevin will be reminded of the rules of free play prior to beginning free play.

**Replacement Behaviors** Kevin will keep his hands and feet to himself during free play.

Kevin will respectfully ask his peers for a toy with school-community-acceptable behavior. (To be taught, but not implemented until he steps down from teacher-controlled toys to sharing toys with peers.)

Kevin will respectfully keep his hands and feet to himself when denied access to a toy from a peer.

Kevin will use self-mediation and self-calming skills, such as taking a deep breath or counting to ten when he is denied access to a tangible item.

**Reinforcers** Token economy—(fixed interval—5 min). A token will represent 2 min. At the end of every 5 min of free play, Kevin has the opportunity to earn an additional 2 min of free time if he uses respectful behavior and does not hit or kick his peers. So, after a 15-min recess, Kevin can earn 0, 2, 4, or 6 extra min of play time to be used later in the day.

Verbal praise and encouragement

After 5 days of success, Kevin will earn a supervised playtime with a peer. This can be supervised by a teacher, paraprofessional, or the school counselor.

**Consequences** Kevin will not earn his token when an infraction occurs.

A social skill mini-lesson will be redelivered regarding sharing, accepting no, and school appropriate behavior.

Communication with parent (note in agenda, e-mail, or phone call depending on severity of behavior)

**Plan of Action** Data will be collected daily by Kevin's teacher on a behavior-monitoring sheet.

Kevin's special education case manager will gather the data weekly and review it.

A behavior-monitoring sheet will be sent home to the parents weekly.

A progress-monitoring report will be sent home as the school system dictates, when all progress reports and report cards are sent home.

Baseline data indicated that Kevin is hitting and kicking during free play 73% of the time. The team will reconvene 1 month after the date of implementation if Kevin has not made 50% progress from his original baseline data.

When Kevin has made 85% progress from his original baseline data, the team will reconvene and discuss continuing the BIP.

Student's name: Kevin Brown

Date: January 25, 2016

Participants: *Milt Scheider, parent*

*Lori Lipscomb, general education teacher*

*Beth K. Sweeten, special education teacher*

*Randall Endor, behavior specialist*

*Felipe R. Anguilar, school counselor*

*Rita Smith, speech language pathologist*

| Target behavior | Function | Modified antecedents | Alternative behaviors | Rewards | Consequences | Action plan |
|---|---|---|---|---|---|---|
| Kevin pushes and kicks other students with his hands and feet during free play, including both in the classroom and on the playground and throughout the school day when free play is given | Kevin's behavior is maintained by the need to gain access to a tangible item (usually a toy) | Social skills training | Kevin will keep his hands and feet to himself during free play | Token economy—(fixed interval—5 min) A token will represent 2 min. At the end of every 5 min of free play, Kevin has the opportunity to earn an additional 2 min of free time if he uses respectful behavior and does not hit or kick his peers. So, after a 15 min recess, Kevin can earn 0, 2, 4, or 6 extra minutes of play time to be used later in the day | Kevin will not earn his token when an infraction occurs | Data will be collected daily by Kevin's teacher on a behavior-monitoring sheet |
| | | Modeling to address sharing and accepting "no" from a peer | Kevin will respectfully ask his peers for a toy with school-community-acceptable behavior. (To be taught, but not implemented until he steps down from teacher-controlled toys to sharing toys with peers.) | Verbal praise and encouragement | A social skill mini-lesson will be redelivered regarding sharing, accepting no, and school-appropriate behavior | Kevin's special education case manager will gather the data weekly and review it |
| | | Prior to free play, allow Kevin to choose three toys that will stay with the teacher for free play. Kevin will have the opportunity to ask the teacher for one of the toys. Then, trade it for another if he chooses throughout free play | Kevin will respectfully keep his hands and feet to himself when denied access to a toy from a peer | After 5 days of success, Kevin will earn a supervised play time with a peer. This can be supervised by a teacher, paraprofessional, or the school counselor | Communication with parent (note in agenda, e-mail, or phone call depending on severity of behavior) | A behavior-monitoring sheet will be sent home to the parents weekly |

| Target behavior | Function | Modified antecedents | Alternative behaviors | Rewards | Consequences | Action plan |
|---|---|---|---|---|---|---|
| | | Kevin will be reminded of the rules of free play prior to beginning free play | Kevin will use self-mediation and self-calming skills, such as taking a deep breath or counting to ten when he is denied access to a tangible item | | | A progress-monitoring report will be sent home as the school system dictates, when all progress reports and report cards are sent home |
| | | | | | | Baseline data indicated that Kevin is hitting and kicking during free play 73 % of the time. The team will reconvene 1 month after the date of implementation if Kevin has not made 50 % progress from his original baseline data |
| | | | | | | When Kevin has made 85 % progress from his original baseline data, the team will reconvene and discuss continuing the behavior intervention plan |

## Strategy Five: What *Not* to Do

1. Do not reinvent the wheel! Use the FBA to inform the BIP.
2. Do not create a BIP without developing an FBA first. (Important, even if it sounds redundant!)
3. Do not confuse consequences and punishments.
4. Do not use reinforcers that are not accessible in the environment.
5. Do not begin without having baseline data.
6. Do not change the plan without current data.

## A Before-You-Proceed Checklist

1. Name and identify the schedules of reinforcements.
2. Understand the difference between consequences and punishments.
3. Know the difference between a skill deficit and a performance deficit.
4. List the components found on a BIP.

**Author Takeaways**

*Takeaway from Stephanie, the behavior specialist*:

There are so many takeaways regarding BIPs. I suppose that I would have two cautionary statements. My first would be in the form of a plea, "Do not think of consequences as a form of punishment!" When we advocate having teachable consequences, we are not saying, "Teach that student a lesson that he will never forget!" We are advocating for the process of decision-making and problem-solving. We are advocating for the adult to teach the student to think through the cause and effect. The second cautionary statement I would make is to utilize the baseline data. Behavior planning is great, but it must be evaluated. We have used the word effectiveness a lot in this chapter. But it is important. If behavior planning is not successful, it needs to be reconsidered. This cannot be done with fidelity if the baseline data gathered in the FBA process are not used.

*Takeaway from Alan, the school psychologist*:

I would have to echo Stephanie's cautionary statements. I also wanted to emphasize that this, like everything else we have discussed in the book, is a process; completing all of this will not happen overnight, and you will not be an expert after completing anything we discussed the first time. As you gain experience completing different components of the FBA, you will find that your skill set is improving. Wherever you work, you may be responsible for only part of the process. A team effort means that not only is the work shared among different professionals, but also different viewpoints and many different skills will be available for completing each step. If the team works collaboratively, a great deal can be done to help students become more successful.

# References

Blair, K. C., Umbreit, J., & Bos, C. S. (1999). Using functional assessment and children's preferences to improve the behavior of young children with behavioral disorders. *Behavioral Disorders, 24*(2), 151–166.

Cipani, E., & Schock, K. M. (2010). *Functional behavioral assessment, diagnosis, and treatment: A complete system for education and mental health settings* (2nd edn.). New York: Springer.

Conroy, M. A., & Stichter, J. P. (2003). The application of antecedents in the functional assessment process: Existing research, issues, and recommendations. *Journal of Special Education, 37*(1), 15–25.

Fad, K. M., Patton, J. R., & Polloway, E. A. (1998). *Behavioral intervention planning: Completing a functional behavioral assessment and developing a behavioral intervention plan.* Austin: PRO–ED.

Gresham, F. M., & Elliott, S. N. (1989). Social skills deficits as a primary learning disability. *Journal of Learning Disabilities, 22*(2), 120–124.

Gresham, F. M., Watson, T. S., & Skinner, C. H. (2001). Functional behavioral assessment: Principles, procedures, and future directions. *School Psychology Review, 30*(2), 156–172.

Jolivette, K., Scott, T. M., & Nelson, C. M. (2000). The link between functional behavior assessments (FBAs) and behavioral intervention plans (BIPs). ERIC Digest, E592, EDO-00-1.

Kern, L., Gallagher, P., Starosta, K., Hickman, W., & George, M. (2006). Longitudinal outcomes of functional behavioral assessment-based intervention. *Journal of Positive Behavior Interventions, 8*(2), 67–78.

Newcomer, L. L., & Lewis, T. J. (2004). Functional behavioral assessment: An investigation of assessment reliability and effectiveness of function-based interventions. *Journal of Emotional and Behavioral Disorders, 12*(3), 168–181.

O'Neill, R. E., Albin, R. W., Storey, K., Horner, R. H., & Sprague, J. R. (2015). *Functional assessment and program development for problem behaviors: A practical handbook* (3rd edn.). Stamford: Cengage.

Scott, T. M., McIntyre, J., Liaupsin, C., Nelson, C. M., Conroy, M., & Payne, L. D. (2005). An examination of the relation between functional behavior assessment and selected intervention strategies with school-based teams. *Journal of Positive Behavior Interventions, 7*(4), 205–215.

Simonsen, B., & Sugai, G. (2013). PBIS in alternative education settings: Positive support for youth with high-risk behavior. *Education and Treatment of Children, 36*(3), 3–14.

# Part V
# Phase IV: Prevention

*Prevention* is the final phase of our multiphasic approach to behavior planning.

**Professional Responsibilities** Within *Prevention,* the practitioner becomes an advocate for a climate of prevention, a culture of prevention, and a community of prevention.

**Alternative View** The *Prevention phase* is not limited to momentary fixes. It is an ongoing effort to create positive environments, which promote positive behavior.

**Task List** With regard to creating a climate of prevention, a culture of prevention, and a community of prevention, the practitioner must:

1. Advocate
2. Lead
3. Plan

**Goal** By the end of this chapter, we hope the practitioner will take the message of prevention into the organizations where they work.

# Chapter 14
# Prevention: Climate, Culture, and Community

## What You Need to Know

*Prevention* is the final phase of our multiphasic approach to behavior planning. Within Prevention, the practitioner not only remains a strong voice but is also a collaborator with the team for the prevention of behaviors. The climate, culture, and community all can equally serve to minimize or increase the demonstration of disruptive behavior. Even with the best *Process, Purpose*, and *Planning* in place, a lack of commitment to *Prevention* as a whole will give rise to behavioral challenges. Without an effort towards prevention, negative and difficult behavior might reemerge despite all other attempts at behavior management.

## *Understanding the Present*

When we began this book, we told you that part of our behavioral philosophy rests on the assumption that behavior cannot be viewed in single, isolated episodes. We shared this idea to remind you that a person's behavior goes beyond one or two occurrences of challenging behavior. We take you back to that now, but with a different expectation of those isolated misconceptions. Interfering behavior does not occur in an isolated vacuum; it occurs within a community. Behavior is learned, and our climate, culture, and community can be some of the strongest teachers. The interfering behavior of one student is the impacting behavior of another.

When we address challenging behavior through Process, Purpose, and Planning, we are intervening for the individual. With Prevention, we need to look beyond the individual to create the climate, culture, and community necessary to build positive organizations. In order to build those organizations, we need to focus on prevention planning.

*Climate* Climate is the atmosphere or the prevailing mood in an organization. Our jobs require us to be in multiple schools, sometimes daily. It is easy to recognize the

© Springer International Publishing Switzerland 2016
S. M. Hadaway, A. W. Brue, *Practitioner's Guide to Functional Behavioral Assessment,*
Autism and Child Psychopathology Series, DOI 10.1007/978-3-319-23721-3_14

prevailing atmosphere when you walk into each separate one. Building a climate of prevention in an organization means creating a climate where individuals want to come—students, residents, and personnel. It is a climate where people feel safe and have a sense of belonging. It is a climate with prevailing positive attitudes towards those around us.

*Culture* Culture is the social norms and collective understanding within an environment. It is the prevailing thought on how things should operate and on how things actually operate. Within our public educational system, there has been an increase in a culture of violence and bullying within our schools. If violence and aggressive behavior are expected in an environment, they will likely continue. Creating a culture of prevention means resetting both the spoken and unspoken expectations that govern environmental behavior.

*Community* Community is a group that shares a common characteristic. Within a workplace, the community is our fellow workers. Within a school, the community is everyone who works, attends, and supports the school. But community can mean so much more than just sharing a characteristic. It can be those interpersonal connections that form and create fellowship, belonging, and loyalty.

## Understanding the Future

In order to create a climate of prevention, a culture, of prevention and a community of prevention, there needs to be planning for both improving the organizational environment and crisis prevention.

Pro-action is necessary in prevention. Simonsen et al. (2014) suggest that schools should consider using something such as Positive Behavior Interventions and Supports (PBIS) to decrease the likelihood and intensity of situations that may need the use of crisis procedures. PBIS is a whole-school prevention strategy that can also help a school prevent disruptive behavior by creating and sustaining a three-tiered system of support, which can improve their ability to respond in an appropriate and accurate manner (Bradshaw et al. 2010). And when used school-wide, PBIS can lead to changes in a school's discipline practices and systems (Barrett et al. 2008; Nersesian et al. 2000; Taylor-Greene and Kartub 2000).

For us, PBIS is at the forefront of proactive strategies that promote prevention, and it is part of the language found in IDEA 2004. Based on ABA principles, PBIS does not just focus on a student with interfering behaviors. Rather, PBIS is a school-wide system of support (Positive Behavioral Interventions and Supports (PBIS) 2014). It focuses on using strategies for defining, teaching, and supporting appropriate student behaviors; and research supports the use of PBIS in general education settings, alternative schools, residential programs, day treatment programs, and juvenile justice facilities (Simonsen and Sugai 2013). The overall approach is to create a positive environment for students to learn, grow, and develop.

However, PBIS cannot just be implemented overnight. It requires planning. This means coming together at all levels and putting into place the system-wide supports necessary for successful execution. It does take effort. Just saying your school has a school-wide rewards program is not enough to actually legitimize PBIS. PBIS requires a far reaching plan that addresses the full range of behaviors and every area in which any of those behaviors occur. The hallway is just as important as the classroom. But, the rewards are well worth it. The overall improvement to climate, culture, and community within the school provides positive results for everyone involved. For more information on PBIS, you can find their website in Appendix B.

Just as planning for improvement is important to prevention, so is planning for the crisis. It is inevitable that at some point a crisis will happen in your organization. Students with interfering behaviors can become dangerous to themselves and to others. The time to decide how to handle a potentially dangerous situation is not as it is happening. Simonsen et al. (2014) note that "Districts should ensure that every educator is (a) familiar with local, state, and federal policies and guidelines related to crisis procedures; (b) aware of their school's/district's operational definition of crisis (i.e., what levels of behavior constitute a crisis); (c) trained to recognize a crisis and request support; and, if appropriate, (d) trained in district-approved crisis response procedures" (p. 315). Good safety and crisis prevention responses require carefully mapping out the strategies and interventions that will be used in an emergency. In the moment of crisis, both staff and the individuals the environment support need to know how to behave in the crisis.

Nationally, there has been a movement to reduce and end restraint and seclusion within institutionalized settings, such as residential programs and schools. Improper restraint has led to lives lost. Yet, we still have to support students and residents who demonstrate highly aggressive and dangerous behavior. So, what do we do?

If one part of your crisis prevention program includes planning, the other part should include training. Both are necessary to create safe environments, and training is especially necessary for intensive supports that require additional skill acquisition occurring beyond typical general classroom management principles (Brunsting et al. 2014). I (Stephanie) first heard the phrase culture of prevention from Marshall M. Siler, the founder of MindSet Consulting, L.L.C. He trains organizations on crisis prevention and physical restraint. The MindSet training curriculum developed by Siler focuses on creating a culture where we prevent escalation. He has identified 12 keys to eliminating and reducing incidents of restraint and seclusion. They are listed below:

- A comprehensive clear policy and procedure
- Restraint must be the intervention of last resort
- Staff must be trained in de-escalation techniques (verbal and visual)
- Adequate and well-prepared staff
- Consumer (student) involvement
- A system of data collection and analysis
- Strategies for organizational change
- Performance measurement systems

- Emphasis on staff and consumer (student) strengths
- Cultural competence
- Effective consumer (student) staff debriefing
- An environment that prioritizes consumer (student) dignity

Organizations that successfully train their staff help to create the prevention needed in their environments. If you do not have a training program, need consulting on crisis prevention, or require further training, we have included MindSet Consulting's contact information in Appendix B under Crisis Prevention Strategies and Physical Restraint Training.

Finally, the climate, culture, and community all can equally serve to minimize or increase the demonstration of disruptive behavior. Prevention is about looking ahead to find those areas where improvement is needed, and then becoming a voice to lead. As we have stated, Process, Purpose, Planning, and Prevention are phases that help us to think about more long-term solutions. As practitioners, it is our hope that these principles will help you work towards prevention in every facet of climate, culture, and community for the individuals you serve and for your organization.

**Author Takeaways**

*Takeaway from Stephanie, the behavior specialist:*

Prevention is perhaps the most important aspect of creating safe environments. All the programs, strategies, and interventions we have discussed are intended to ultimately guide you towards prevention. It has been my experience that students at risk do not typically thrive in unstable and chaotic environments. They succeed in consistent, positive environments where the rules are understandable and applicable. Inconsistency is a breeding ground for negative behavior. Establishing PBIS within your school helps to create an environment where the right types of behaviors are reinforced. Training your staff in de-escalation programs, like MindSet, helps to further establish stability in environments that can sometimes become unstable. Using your resources to develop adequate behavior plans at the individual and even school level might seem like a big undertaking. But, my guess is that you already do this on some level every day. Supporting students or residents with interfering, challenging, or problem behaviors by developing functional behavioral assessments (FBAs) is a process that leads you to the purpose of the behavior which in turn allows you to plan in the hopes of preventing future behaviors. I hope that you will use the plans we have discussed in this book. It might be challenging at first, but it will get easier in time.

*Takeaway from Alan, the school psychologist:*

We hope that you will find our approach useful in your work. An FBA can be a very helpful tool. Knowing how to conduct one—and to do so correctly—is important so that the information you collect is reliable and valid. Do not hesitate to go back and read through specific chapters again. You may be unfamiliar with certain concepts and may find them difficult to understand. Once you move beyond theory and put this information into practice, I think you will find it more easily digestible. Like anything else, it can take practice to be confident in your ability to do an FBA and behavioral intervention plan (BIP) correctly. Should you need additional information, do not forget to use the resources we listed in Appendix B.

## References

Barrett, S. B., Bradshaw, C. P., & Lewis-Palmer, T. (2008). Maryland statewide PBIS initiative: Systems, evaluation, and next steps. *Journal of Positive Behavior Interventions, 10*(2), 105–114.

Bradshaw, C., Mitchell, M., & Leaf, P. (2010). Examining the effects of school-wide positive behavioral interventions and supports on student outcomes: Results from a randomized controlled effectiveness trial in elementary schools. *Journal of Positive Behavior Interventions, 12,* 133–148.

Brunsting, N. C., Sreckovic, M. A., & Lane, K. L. (2014). Special education teacher burnout: A synthesis of research from 1979 to 2013. *Education and Treatment of Children, 37*(4), 681–711.

Nersesian, M., Todd, A., Lehmann, J., & Watson, J. (2000). School- wide behavior support through district-level system change. *Journal of Positive Behavior Interventions, 2*(4), 244–247.

Positive Behavioral Interventions and Supports (PBIS). (2014, August 20). SWPBIS for beginners. Retrieved from http://www.pbis.org/school/swpbis-for-beginners.

Simonsen, B., & Sugai, G. (2013). PBIS in alternative education settings: Positive support for youth with high-risk behavior. *Education and Treatment of Children, 36*(3), 3–14.

Simonsen, B., Sugai, G., Freeman, J., Kern, L., & Hampton, J. (2014). Ethical and professional guidelines for use of crisis procedures. *Education and Treatment of Children, 37*(2), 307–322.

Taylor-Greene, S. J., & Kartub, D. T. (2000). Durable implementation of school-wide behavior support: The high five program. *Journal of Positive Behavior Interventions, 2*(4), 233–235.

# Appendices

## Appendix A

### *State Contact Information*

Below is the contact information for each state's Department of Education and Office of Special Education. Contact them with any questions you may have about the policies and procedures in your state.

*Alabama*
Alabama Department of Education
P.O. Box 302101
50 North Ripley Street
Montgomery, AL 36104–3833
Phone: (334) 242-9700
Fax: (334) 242-9708
Website: http://www.alsde.edu/Pages/home.aspx

Special Education Services
Alabama State Department of Education
P.O. Box 302101
Montgomery, AL 36130-2101
Phone: (334) 242-8114
Toll-Free: (800) 392-8020 AL residents only
Fax: (334) 242-9192
Website: http://www.alsde.edu/sec/ses/Pages/home.aspx

*Alaska*
Alaska Department of Education and Early Development
801 West 10th Street, Suite 200
P.O. Box 110500

© Springer International Publishing Switzerland 2016
S. M. Hadaway, A. W. Brue, *Practitioner's Guide to Functional Behavioral Assessment,*
Autism and Child Psychopathology Series, DOI 10.1007/978-3-319-23721-3

Juneau, AK 99811-0500
Phone: (907) 465-2800
Fax: (907) 465-4156
Website: http://www.eed.state.ak.us/

Special Education Office
Alaska State Department of Education and Early Development
801 West 10th Street, Suite 200
P.O. Box 110500
Juneau, AK 99811-0500
Phone: (907) 465-8693
Fax: (907) 465-2806
Website: http://www.eed.state.ak.us/tls/sped/home.html

***Arizona***
Arizona Department of Education
1535 West Jefferson Street
Phoenix, AZ 85007
Phone: (602) 542-4361
Toll-Free: (800) 352-4558
Fax: (602) 542-5440
Website: http://www.ade.az.gov/

Exceptional Student Services
Arizona State Department of Education
3300 N. Central Avenue
Phoenix, AZ 85007
Phone: (602) 542-4013
Toll-Free: (800) 352-4558 AZ residents only
Fax: (602) 542-5404
Website: http://www.ade.state.az.us/ess/

***Arkansas***
Arkansas Department of Education
Four State Capitol Mall
Little Rock, AR 72201-1071
Phone: (501) 682-4475
Fax: (501) 682-1079
Website: http://www.arkansased.org/

Special Education Services
Arkansas State Department of Education
Victory Building, Suite 450
1401 West Capitol Avenue
Little Rock, AR 72201-2936

Phone: (501) 682-4221
Fax: (501) 682-5159
Website: http://arksped.k12.ar.us/

*California*
California Department of Education
1430 N. Street
Sacramento, CA 95814-5901
Phone: (916) 319-0800
Fax: (916) 319-0100
Website: http://www.cde.ca.gov/

Special Education Division
California State Department of Education
1430 N. Street, Suite 2401
Sacramento, CA 95814-5901
Phone: (916) 445-4613
Fax: (916) 327-3706
Website: http://www.cde.ca.gov/sp/se/

*Colorado*
Colorado Department of Education
201 East Colfax Avenue
Denver, CO 80203-1704
Phone: (303) 866-6600
Fax: (303) 830-0793
Website: http://www.cde.state.co.us/

Exceptional Student Leadership Unit
Colorado State Department of Education
1560 Broadway, Suite 1175
Denver, CO 80202
Phone: (303) 866-6694
Fax: (303) 866-6767
Website: http://www.cde.state.co.us/cdesped/index.asp

*Connecticut*
Connecticut Department of Education
165 Capitol Avenue
Hartford, CT 06106-1630
Phone: (860) 713-6543
Toll-Free: (800) 465-4014
Fax: (860) 713-7001
Website: http://www.sde.ct.gov/

Bureau of Special Education
Connecticut State Department of Education
Room 369
P.O. Box 2219
Hartford, CT 06145-2219
Phone: (860) 713-6912
Fax: (860) 713-7014
Website: http://www.sde.ct.gov/sde/cwp/view.asp?a=2678&Q=320730

### *Delaware*
Delaware Department of Education
The Townsend Building
401 Federal Street, Suite 2
Dover, DE 19901-3639
Phone: (302) 735-4000
Fax: (302) 739-4654
Website: http://www.doe.k12.de.us/

Exceptional Children and Early Childhood Education
Delaware Department of Education
401 Federal Street, Suite 2
Dover, DE 19901-3639
Phone: (302) 735-4210
Fax: (302) 739-2388
Website: http://www.doe.k12.de.us/Page/183

### *District of Columbia*
Office of the State Superintendent of Education
801 1st Street NE, 9th Floor
Washington, DC 20002
Phone: (202) 727-6436
Fax: (202) 727-2019
Website: http://osse.dc.gov/

DCPS Office of Specialized Instruction
1200 First Street, NE, 9th Floor
Washington, DC 20002
Phone: (202) 442-4800
Website: http://dcps.dc.gov/DCPS/In+the+Classroom/Special+Education

### *Florida*
Florida Department of Education
325 West Gaines Street
Tallahassee, FL 32399-0400
Phone: (850) 245-0505

Fax: (850) 245-9667
Website: http://www.fldoe.org/

Florida Department of Education
Bureau of Exceptional Education and Student Services
325 West Gaines Street
Tallahassee, FL 32399-0400
Phone: (850) 245-0475
Fax: (850) 245-0953
Website: http://www.fldoe.org/academics/exceptional-student-edu/

*Georgia*
Georgia Department of Education
205 Jesse Hill Jr. Drive, SE
Atlanta, GA 30334-5001
Phone: (404) 656-2800
Toll-Free: (800) 311-3627 GA residents only
Fax: (404) 651-8737
Website: http://www.gadoe.org

Georgia Department of Education
Division for Special Education Services and Supports
205 Jesse Hill Jr. Drive SE
Atlanta, GA 30334
Phone: (404) 656-3963
Fax: (404) 651-6457
Website: http://public.doe.k12.ga.us/ci_exceptional.aspx

*Hawaii*
Hawaii Department of Education
1390 Miller Street
Honolulu, HI 96813
Phone: (808) 586-3230
Website: http://www.hawaiipublicschools.org/Pages/home.aspx

Hawaii State Department of Education
Special Education Section
475 22nd Avenue
Building 302, Room 115
Honolulu, HI 96816
Phone: (808) 733-4400
Toll-Free: (800) 297-2070
Fax: (808) 733-4841
Website: http://www.hawaiipublicschools.org/TeachingAndLearning/Specialized-Programs/SpecialEducation/Pages/home.aspx

## *Idaho*

Idaho State Board of Education
650 West State Street
Boise, ID 83720-0027
Phone: (208) 332-6800
Fax: (208) 334-2228
Website: http://www.sde.idaho.gov/

Idaho State Department of Education
Division of Special Education
P.O. Box 83720
Boise, ID 83720-0047
Toll-Free: (800) 432-4601
Fax: (208) 334-2228
Website: http://www.sde.idaho.gov/site/special_edu/

## *Illinois*

Illinois State Board of Education
100 North First Street
Springfield, IL 62777
Phone: (217) 782-4321
Toll-Free: (866) 262-6663 IL residents only
Fax: (217) 524-4928
Website: http://www.isbe.net/

Illinois State Board of Education
100 North First Street
Springfield, IL 62777-0001
Phone: (217) 782-5589
Fax: (217) 782-9224
Website: http://www.isbe.net/spec-ed/

## *Indiana*

Indiana Department of Education
South Tower, Suite 600
115 W. Washington Street
Indianapolis, IN 46204-2795
Phone: (317) 232-6610
Fax: (317) 232-6610
Website: http://www.doe.in.gov

Indiana Department of Education
Office of Special Education
South Tower, Suite 600
115 W. Washington Street

Indianapolis, IN 46204
Phone: (317) 232-0570
Toll-Free: (877) 851-4106
Fax: (317) 232-0589
Website: http://www.doe.in.gov/specialed

*Iowa*
Iowa Department of Education
Grimes State Office Building
400 East 14th Street
Des Moines, IA 50319-0146
Phone: (515) 281-5294
Fax: (515) 242-5988
Website: http://educateiowa.gov

Bureau of Learner Strategies and Supports
Iowa Department of Education
Grimes State Office Building
400 East 14th Street
Des Moines, IA 50319-0146
Phone: (515) 281-5294
Fax: (515) 242-5988
Website: https://www.educateiowa.gov/pk-12/special-education

*Kansas*
Kansas Department of Education
Landon State Office Building
900 SW Jackson Street
Topeka, KS 66612-1212
Phone: (785) 296-3201
Website: http://www.ksde.org/

Special Education Services
Kansas State Department of Education
900 SW Jackson Street
Topeka, KS 66612
Phone: (785) 296-9462
Toll-Free: (800) 203-9462 KS Residents only
Website: http://www.ksde.org/Default.aspx?tabid=506

*Kentucky*
Kentucky Department of Education
Capital Plaza Tower
500 Metro Street
Frankfort, KY 40601

Phone: (502) 564-3141
Website: http://www.education.ky.gov

Special Education Services
Kentucky Department of Education
500 Metro Street, 18 Floor CPT
Frankfort, KY 40601
Phone: (502) 564-4970
Fax: (502) 564-6721
Website: http://education.ky.gov/specialed/excep/Pages/default.aspx

*Louisiana*
Louisiana Department of Education
1201 North Third Street
Baton Rouge, LA 70804-9064
Toll-Free: (877) 453-2721
Fax: (225) 342-0193
Website: http://www.louisianabelieves.com/

Louisiana Department of Education
Office of Student Programs
Division of NCLB and IDEA Support
P.O. Box 94064
Baton Rouge, LA 7804
Phone: (225) 219-0364
Toll-Free: (877) 453-2721
Fax: (225) 219-7370
Website: http://www.louisianabelieves.com/academics/students-with-disabilities

*Maine*
Maine Department of Education
23 State House Station
Augusta, ME 04333-0023
Phone: (207) 624-6600
Fax: (207) 624-6601
Website: http://www.maine.gov/doe/

Office of Special Services
Maine Department of Education
23 State House Station
Augusta, ME 04333-0023
Phone: (207) 624-6676
Fax: (207) 624-6651
TTY: 1-888-577-6690
Website: http://www.maine.gov/education/speced/index.htm

*Maryland*
Maryland State Department of Education
200 West Baltimore Street
Baltimore, MD 21201
Phone: (410) 767-0100
Fax: (410) 333-6033
Website: http://www.marylandpublicschools.org

Division of Special Education/Early Intervention Services
Maryland State Department of Education
200 West Baltimore Street
Baltimore, MD 21201
Phone: (410) 767-0238
Toll-Free: (800) 535-0182
Fax: (410) 333-8165
Website: http://www.marylandpublicschools.org/MSDE/divisions/earlyinterv/

*Massachusetts*
Massachusetts Department of Elementary and Secondary Education
75 Pleasant Street
Malden, MA 02148-4906
Phone: (781) 338-3102
Fax: (781) 338-3770
Website: http://www.doe.mass.edu/

Special Education Planning and Policy Development Office
State Department of Elementary and Secondary Education
75 Pleasant Street
Malden, MA 02148-5023
Phone: (781) 338-3375
Fax: (781) 338-3371
Website: http://www.doe.mass.edu/sped/

*Michigan*
Michigan Department of Education
608 West Allegan Street
P.O. Box 30008
Lansing, MI 48909
Phone: (517) 373-3324
Website: http://www.michigan.gov/mde/

Office of Special Education and Early Intervention Services
Michigan Department of Education
608 West Allegan Street
P.O. Box 30008

Lansing, MI 48909
Phone: (517) 373-3324
Website: https://www.michigan.gov/mde/0,4615,7-140-6530_6598--,00.html

*Minnesota*
Minnesota Department of Education
1500 Highway 36 West
Roseville, MN 55113-4266
Phone: (651) 582-8200
Website: http://education.state.mn.us/mde/index.html

Special Education Division
Minnesota State Department of Education
1500 Highway 36 West
Roseville, MN 55113-4266
Phone: (651) 582-8614
Fax: (651) 582-8729
Website: http://education.state.mn.us/MDE/EdExc/SpecEdClass

*Mississippi*
Mississippi Department of Education
P.O. Box 771
Jackson, MS 39205
Phone: (601) 359-3513
Website: http://www.mde.k12.ms.us/

Office of Special Education
Mississippi State Department of Education
359 North West Street, Suite 301
P.O. Box 771
Jackson, MS 39205-0771
Phone: (601) 359-3498
Toll-Free: (877) 544-0408 MS residents only
Website: http://www.mde.k12.ms.us/special-education

*Missouri*
Missouri Department of Elementary and Secondary Education
205 Jefferson Street
Jefferson City, MO 65102-0480
Phone: (573) 751-4212
Fax: (573) 751-8613
Website: http://dese.mo.gov/

Division of Special Education
Missouri State Department of Elementary and Secondary Education

205 Jefferson Street
P.O. Box 480
Jefferson City, MO 65101
Phone: (573) 751-5739
Website: http://dese.mo.gov/special-education

### Montana

Montana Office of Public Instruction
P.O. Box 202501
Helena, MT 59620-2501
Phone: (406) 444-2082
Toll-Free: (888) 231-9393 (Area code 406 only)
Fax: (406) 444-3924
Website: http://www.opi.mt.gov/

Division of Special Education
Montana State Office of Public Instruction
P.O. Box 202501
Helena, MT 59620-2501
Phone: (406) 444-3095
Website: http://www.opi.mt.gov/Programs/SpecialEd/

### Nebraska

Nebraska Department of Education
301 Centennial Mall South
P.O. Box 94987
Lincoln, NE 68509
Phone: (402) 471-2295
Fax: 402-471-4433
Website: http://www.education.ne.gov

Office of Special Education
Nebraska State Department of Education
301 Centennial Mall South
P.O. Box 94987
Lincoln, NE 68509-4987
Phone: (402) 471-2471
Fax: (402) 471-5022
Website: http://www.education.ne.gov/sped/index.html

### Nevada

Nevada Department of Education
700 East Fifth Street
Carson City, NV 89701
Phone: (775) 687-9200

Fax: (775) 687-9101
Website: http://www.doe.nv.gov/

Office of Special Education
Nevada State Department of Education
700 East Fifth Street
Carson City, NV 89701
Phone: (775) 687-9200
Fax: (775) 687-9101
Website: http://www.doe.nv.gov/Office_of_Special_Education/

*New Hampshire*
New Hampshire Department of Education
101 Pleasant Street
Concord, NH 03301
Phone: (603) 271-3494
Website: http://www.ed.state.nh.us

Bureau of Special Education
New Hampshire Department of Education
101 Pleasant Street
Concord, NH 03301
Phone: (603) 271-3494
Website: http://www.education.nh.gov/instruction/special_ed/index.htm

*New Jersey*
New Jersey Department of Education
100 Riverview Plaza
P.O. Box 500
Trenton, NJ 08625-0500
Phone: (609) 292-4450
Fax: (609) 777-4099
Website: http://www.state.nj.us/education/

Office of Special Education Programs
New Jersey Department of Education
P.O. Box 500
Trenton, NJ 08625-0500
Phone: (609) 292-0147
TTY: (609) 984-8422
Website: http://www.nj.gov/njded/specialed/

*New Mexico*
New Mexico Public Education Department
300 Don Gaspar Avenue

Santa Fe, NM 87501
Phone: (505) 827-5800
Website: http://ped.state.nm.us/ped/index.html

New Mexico Public Education Department
Special Education Bureau
120 South Federal Place, Room 206
Santa Fe, NM 87501
Phone: (505) 827-1457
Fax: (505) 954-0001
Website: http://www.ped.state.nm.us/seo/index.htm

*New York*
New York State Education Department
89 Washington Avenue
Albany, NY 12234
Phone: (518) 474-3852
Website: http://www.nysed.gov/

P-12: Office of Special Education
New York State Education Department
89 Washington Avenue, Room 309 EB
One Commerce Plaza
Albany, NY 12234
Phone: (518) 474-3852
Website: http://www.p12.nysed.gov/specialed/

*North Carolina*
North Carolina Department of Public Instruction
301 North Wilmington Street
Raleigh, NC 27601
Phone: (919) 807-3300
Website: http://www.ncpublicschools.org/

Exceptional Children Division
North Carolina Department of Public Instruction
6356 Mail Service Center
Raleigh, NC 27699-6356
Phone: (919) 807-3969
Website: http://ec.ncpublicschools.gov/

*North Dakota*
North Dakota Department of Public Instruction
Department 201
600 East Boulevard Avenue

Bismarck, ND 58505-0440
Phone: (701) 328-2260
Website: http://www.dpi.state.nd.us

Office of Special Education
North Dakota State Department of Public Instruction
Department 201
600 East Boulevard Avenue
Bismarck, ND 58505-0440
Phone: (701) 328-2277
Website: http://www.dpi.state.nd.us/speced1/index.shtm

### Ohio
Ohio Department of Education
25 South Front Street
Columbus, OH 43215-4183
Toll-Free: (877) 644-6338
Website: http://www.ode.state.oh.us/

Office for Exceptional Children
Ohio Department of Education
25 South Front Street, Mail Stop 409
Columbus, OH 43215-4183
Phone: (614) 466-2650
Toll-Free: (877) 644-6338
Fax: (614) 387-0968
Website: http://education.ohio.gov/Topics/Special-Education

### Oklahoma
Oklahoma State Department of Education
Oliver Hodge Building
2500 North Lincoln Boulevard
Oklahoma City, OK 73105-4599
Phone: (405) 521-3301
Fax: (405) 521-6938
Website: http://www.ok.gov/sde/
Special Education Services

Oklahoma State Department of Education
Oliver Hodge Building
2500 North Lincoln Boulevard
Oklahoma City, OK 73105-4599
Phone: (405) 521-4862
Website: http://www.ok.gov/sde/special-education

## Oregon
Oregon Department of Education
255 Capitol Street, NE
Salem, OR 97310-0203
Phone: (503) 947-5600
Fax: (503) 378-5156
Website: http://www.ode.state.or.us/home/

Office of Special Education
Oregon State Department of Education
255 Capitol Street, NE
Salem, OR 97310-0203
Phone: (503) 947-5600
Website: http://www.ode.state.or.us/search/page/?id=2901

## Pennsylvania
Pennsylvania Department of Education
333 Market Street
Harrisburg, PA 17126-0333
Phone: (717) 783-6788
Website: http://www.pde.state.pa.us/

Bureau of Special Education
Pennsylvania State Department of Education
333 Market Street
Harrisburg, PA 17126-0333
Phone: (717) 783-6913
Website: http://www.portal.state.pa.us/portal/server.pt/community/special_education/7465

## Rhode Island
Rhode Island Department of Education
255 Westminster Street
Providence, RI 02903-3400
Phone: (401) 222-4600
Website: http://www.ride.ri.gov/

Office for Special Education
Rhode Island Department of Education
255 Westminster Street
Providence, RI 02903-3400
Phone: (401) 222-4600
Website: http://www.ride.ri.gov/StudentsFamilies/SpecialEducation.aspx

### South Carolina
South Carolina Department of Education
1006 Rutledge Building
1429 Senate Street
Columbia, SC 29201
Phone: (803) 734-8500
Website: http://ed.sc.gov/

Office of Special Education
South Carolina State Department of Education
1006 Rutledge Building
1429 Senate Street
Columbia, SC 29201
Phone: (803) 734-8224
Fax: (803) 734-5021
Website: http://ed.sc.gov/agency/ccr/Special-Education-Services/

### South Dakota
South Dakota Department of Education
800 Governors Drive
Pierre, SD 57501-2291
Phone: (605) 773-3134
Website: http://doe.sd.gov/
Special Education Programs

South Dakota State Department of Education
306 East Capitol Avenue, Suite 200
Pierre, SD 57501-2545
Phone: (605) 773-3455
Fax: (605) 773-5320
Website: http://doe.sd.gov/oess/sped.aspx

### Tennessee
Tennessee State Department of Education
710 James Robertson Parkway
Nashville, TN 37243-0375
Phone: (615) 741-5158
Website: http://www.state.tn.us/education/

Tennessee State Department of Education
Special Education Department
710 James Robertson Parkway
Nashville, TN 37243-0375
Phone: (615) 741-5158
Website: http://www.state.tn.us/education/student_support/special_education.shtml

## *Texas*
Texas Education Agency
1701 North Congress Avenue
Austin, TX 78701-1494
Phone: (512) 463-9734
Website: http://www.tea.state.tx.us/

Texas Education Agency
Office of Special Education
1701 North Congress Avenue
Austin, TX 78701-1494
Phone: (512) 463-9734
Website:      http://tea.texas.gov/Curriculum_and_Instructional_Programs/Special_
Education/

## *Utah*
Utah State Office of Education
250 East 500 South
P.O. Box 144200
Salt Lake City, UT 84114-4200
Phone: (801) 538-7500
Website: http://www.schools.utah.gov

Special Education Services
Utah State Office of Education
250 East 500 South
P.O. Box 144200
Salt Lake City, UT 84114-4200
Phone: (801) 538-7500
Website: http://www.schools.utah.gov/sars/

## *Vermont*
Vermont Agency of Education
219 North Main Street, Suite 402
Barre, VT 05641
Phone: (802) 479-1030
Website: http://www.education.vermont.gov/

Office of Special Education
219 North Main Street, Suite 402
Barre, VT 05641
Phone: (802) 479-1030
Website: http://education.vermont.gov/special-education

*Virginia*
Virginia Department of Education
James Monroe Building
101 North 14th Street
Richmond, VA 23218-2120
Phone: (804) 786-7082
Website: http://www.doe.virginia.gov/

Office of Special Education
Virginia State Department of Education
James Monroe Building
101 North 14th Street
Richmond, VA 23218-2120
Phone: (804) 486-8079
Website: http://www.doe.virginia.gov/special_ed/index.shtml

*Washington*
Office of Superintendent of Public Instruction
Old Capitol Building
600 South Washington
P.O. Box 47200
Olympia, WA 98504-7200
Phone: (360) 725-6000
Website: http://www.k12.wa.us/

Special Education Programs
Washington Office of Superintendent of Public Instruction
Old Capitol Building
600 South Washington
P.O. Box 47200
Olympia, WA 98504-7200
Phone: (360) 725-6075
Website: http://www.k12.wa.us/specialed/

*West Virginia*
West Virginia Department of Education
1900 Kanawha Boulevard East
Charleston, WV 25305-0330
Phone: (304) 558-2681
Website: http://wvde.state.wv.us/

Office of Special Education
West Virginia Department of Education
1900 Kanawha Boulevard East
Charleston, WV 25305-0330

Phone: (304) 558-2681
Website: http://wvde.state.wv.us/institutional/SpecialEd/SpecialEdMainPage.html

*Wisconsin*
Wisconsin Department of Public Instruction
125 South Webster Street
P.O. Box 7841
Madison, WI 53707-7841
Phone: (608) 266-3390
Toll-Free: (800) 441-4563
Website: http://dpi.wi.gov/

Special Education Team
Wisconsin Department of Public Instruction
125 South Webster Street
P.O. Box 7841
Madison, WI 53707-7841
Phone: (608) 266-1781
Website: http://sped.dpi.wi.gov/

*Wyoming*
Wyoming Department of Education
Hathaway Building, Second Floor
2300 Capitol Avenue
Cheyenne, WY 82002-0050
Phone: (307) 777-7675
Fax: (307) 777-6234
Website: http://edu.wyoming.gov/

Special Programs Unit
Wyoming State Department of Education
Hathaway Building, Second Floor
2300 Capitol Avenue
Cheyenne, WY 82002-0050
Phone: (307) 777-7675
Fax: (307) 777-6234
Website: http://edu.wyoming.gov/in-the-classroom/special-programs/

# Appendix B

## *Helpful Resources*

Below is a list of resources for books, websites and professional organizations that will be helpful in all stages of behavior planning.

**Books**

*The Complete Guide to Special Education: Expert Advice on Evaluations, IEPs, and Helping Kids Succeed (2nd ed.)* by Linda Wilmshurst and Alan W. Brue (Jossey-Bass, 2010). ISBN: 978-0470615157.

*Incredible Flexible You Deluxe Curriculum Set* by Ryan Hendrix, Kari Zweber Palmer, Nancy Tarshis, and Michelle Garcia Winner (Think Social, 2013). ISBN: 978-1936943050.

*Practical Ideas that Really Work for Students with Disruptive, Defiant, or Difficult Behaviors: Grade 5 through Grades 12 (2nd ed.)* by Kathleen McConnell, Gail Ryser, & James R. Patton (ProEd, 2010). ISBN: 978-1416404606.

*Practical Ideas that Really Work for Students with Disruptive, Defiant, or Difficult Behaviors: Preschool through Grade 4 (2nd ed.)* by Kathleen McConnell, Gail Ryser, & James R. Patton (ProEd, 2010). ISBN: 978-1416404637.

*Self-Regulation for Kids K-12: Strategies for Calming Minds and Behavior* by Patricia Tollison, Katherine O. Synatschk, and Gaea Logan (ProEd, 2010). ISBN: 978-1416404835.

*Superflex... A Superhero Social Thinking Curriculum* by Stephanie Madrigal and Michelle Garcia Winner (Think Social, 2008). ISBN: 978-0979292248.

*Think Social!* by Michelle Garcia Winner (Think Social, 2006). ISBN: 978-0970132048.

*Thinking About You, Thinking About Me (2nd ed.)* by Michelle Garcia Winner (Think Social, 2007). ISBN: 978-0970132062.

*Understanding and Teaching Emotionally Disturbed Children and Adolescents* by Phyllis L. Newcomer (ProEd, 2011). ISBN: 978-1416404910.

*Whole Body Listening Larry at Home* by Kristen Wilson and Elizabeth Sautter (Think Social, 2011). ISBN: 978-0982523179.

*Whole Body Listening Larry at School* by Kristen Wilson and Elizabeth Sautter (Think Social, 2011). ISBN: 978-0982523186.

*You are a Social Detective* by Michelle Garcia Winner and Pamela Crooke (Think Social, 2008). ISBN: 978-0979292262.

*Zones of Regulation* by Leah Kuypers (Think Social, 2011). ISBN: 978-0982523162.

**Crisis Prevention Strategies and Physical Restraint Training**
MindSet Consulting, L.L.C.
18 Mt Vernon Circle
Asheville, NC 28804
Phone: 828-775-5054
Website: http://www.mindsetconsulting.net/

**Internet Sites**
Alan W. Brue, Ph.D.
Website: http://www.alanbrue.com

Center for Effective Collaboration and Practice
Functional Behavioral Assessment
Website: http://cecp.air.org/fba/

Individuals with Disabilities Education Improvement Act of 2004
Website: http://idea.ed.gov

Positive Behavioral Interventions & Supports (PBIS)
https://www.pbis.org

University of Kansas
Functional Behavioral Assessment
Website:    http://www.specialconnections.ku.edu/~kucrl/cgi-bin/drupal/?q=behavior_
plans/functional_behavior_assessment

**Organizations**
The Council for Exceptional Children
Resources for the Public
Website: http://www.cec.sped.org

National Association of School Psychologists
Information for Educators
Website: http://www.nasponline.org/educators/index.aspx

National Association of Special Education Teachers
Resources for Teachers
Website: http://www.naset.org

National Board for Certified Counselors
Resources for the Public
Website: http://www.nbcc.org/PublicResources

U.S. Department of Education
Office of Special Education and Rehabilitative Services
Website: http://www2.ed.gov/about/offices/list/osers/index.html

U.S. Department of Education
Office of Special Education and Rehabilitative Services' Office of Special Education Programs
http://www2.ed.gov/about/offices/list/osers/osep/index.html

# Appendix C

**Functional Behavioral Assessment**
**Phase One: Process**
**Target Behavior Help Sheet**

**Student Name:** _____          **Date:**_____

Identify One to Three Target Behaviors. They need to be specific and measurable. Ask these questions. Write in any that apply. Include substantiating data (record reviews, observation, etc.)

1) What behaviors are most intense? _____
2) What behaviors are most frequent? _____
3) What behaviors have the longest duration? _____
4) Which behaviors are most atypical? _____
5) Which behaviors are the most inappropriate? _____
6) Which behaviors are the most interfering? _____
7) Which behaviors are the most uncontrolled? _____
8) Which behaviors are the most dangerous?_____

**Avoid Vague Descriptions:**

| | | | |
|---|---|---|---|
| Aggressive | Disruptive | Tantrums | Outbursts |
| Inattentive | Off-task | Feeling Words | Avoids |
| Psychotic | Hyperactive | Destructive | Upset |

**What does the behavior look like? Ask the following:**

1. Who?_____
2. What?_____
3. When?_____
And sometimes…
4. How?_____

**Target Behavior Example: Too Vague:** Carla is disruptive in reading.
**Ask:** How is she disruptive? What does her disruptive behavior look like? With whom is she disruptive? When does this disruption occur?
**Target Behavior**: Carla talks out both on and off topic to her teacher throughout her reading lessons.

**Target Behavior One:** _____

**Target Behavior Two:** _____

**Target Behavior Three:** _____

# Appendix D

**Functional Behavioral Assessment**
**Phase One: Process**
**Parent/Caregiver Questionnaire**

**Student/Resident/Individual Name:** _____**Date:** _____
**Parents/Caregivers Present (Name and Relationship to Student/Resident/Individual):**

_____

_____

_____

**Target Behavior(s):** _____

_____

Please use the individual's name in the place of student/resident/individual.

Warm Up Questions: In this first phase of the interview, focus on more neutral topics. The information in the warm up questions can be revisited in Phase Three: Planning.

**Relationships:**

1) Please describe your relationship with the student/resident/individual. _____

_____

2) Who lives in the home with the student/resident/individual? _____

_____

3) Does he/she have any siblings? If so, what are their ages? Do they live in the home? ____

_____

4) Does the student/resident/individual get along with siblings? Describe._____

_____

5) Are there any family members that the student/resident/individual does not get along well

with? Describe. _____

_____

6) Are there any family members with whom the student/resident/individual has a special bond

or enjoys being around? Describe. _____

_____

**Routines:**

7) What is a typical day like with him/her? _____

_____

8) Does he/she have any chores or household responsibilities? If so, what are they? _____

_____

9) Does he/she begin and/or complete the chores when prompted? Or, do chores become difficult due to his/her behaviors?_____

_____

10) Does he/she have a set bedtime? If yes, what time? _____

11) Does he/she go to bed when prompted? Or, does bedtime become difficult due to his/her

behaviors? _____

_____

12) Are there any other routines or activities that the student is required to attend or participate in? Do these become difficult due to his/her behaviors? _____

_____

**Attributes:**

13) Given what you know about the student/resident/individual of him/her, would you please name some of his/her favorite things to do? (ex.,Games, Activities, Talents, Sports, Interests)

_____

14) Name some qualities about him/her. (ex., Friendly, Outgoing, Loyal, Honest, Compassionate) _____

_____

15) Are there any awards or achievements that he/she has received? (ex., Honor Roll, Sports Recognition, Chorus Recognition) _____

_____

**Target Behavior Questions:** In this phase of the interview, focus on the target behavior. If there are other behaviors that seem to be more pervasive or challenging in the environment, be sure to investigate these as well.

16) **Characteristics:** Describe the act or actions that the student/resident/individual exhibits that are interfering, disruptive or problematic. Which behaviors seem to be atypical, inappropriate, interfering, uncontrolled, and/or dangerous? If the person being interviewed uses vague descriptions (aggressive, emotion words) redirect and ask them to describe the behavior (hits with fist, runs from classroom, yells verbal threats, such as "I'll kill you!") _____

_____

_____

_____

_____

17) **Pervasiveness:** Tell me more about the student's/resident's/individual's behavior. Prompt questions for clarification: How frequently does the behavior occur? (This can range from multiple times in an hour to monthly.) How intense is the behavior? (This can range from mildly disruptive to causing physical injury to someone.) Finally, what is the duration of the behavior? (This can range from a few seconds to ongoing throughout the entire day.) If there is more than one target behavior, gather this data on each of the behaviors. _____

_____

_____

_____

**Environmental Conditions:** Tell me more about the environmental factors that surround these behavior(s).

18) Where does the behavior occur? What is the setting? (ex., inside the house, in the community, at church, in the living or common area of the home, at a neighbor's house) _____

_____

_____

19) Is there any place that he/she does not like to be? Is there a place that angers or frightens the student/resident/individual? _____

_____

_____

20) Is there any place that he/she likes to be? Is there a place that the student/resident/individual enjoys or looks forward to attending? _____

_____

_____

21) Who is present when the behavior occurs? (ex., parents, stepparents, siblings, step-siblings, grandparents, other family members, neighbors, and/or strangers) _____

_____

_____

22) Is there anyone he/she likes to be around? Who are his/her friends? _____

_____

_____

23) Does anyone trigger the student's/resident's/individual's behavior? Provoke the behavior?

_____

_____

_____

24) When does the behavior occur? (ex., morning, afternoon, a specific time, or even a specific season) _____

_____

_____

25) Is there a time when the behavior never occurs? (ex., morning, afternoon, a specific time, or even a specific season) _____

_____

26) What is typically happening when this behavior(s) occurs? What are the events or activities taking place? (ex., chores, bed/bath-time, sports, playing games) _____

_____

_____

27) What types of activities or events does the student/resident/individual enjoy? _____

_____

_____

28) What types of activities or events does the student/resident/individual dislike? _____

_____

_____

29) What other triggers can you think of that prompt the behavior of concern? _____

_____

_____

**Respondent Conditions:** The student or resident is considered the respondent.

30) Are there any past or current physiological factors that the student/resident/individual has or is experiencing? (ex., mental health issues, illnesses, genetic disorders, chronic conditions and/or other types of impairments or difficulties) _____

_____

_____

31) For a moment, please consider the student/resident/individual. Are there any cultural considerations we should consider? Has he/she always lived in this country? State? Region? Are there any other social rituals, beliefs, language areother differences that he/she experiences?

_____

_____

_____

32) Are there any pharmacological factors that should be considered? Is the student receiving prescribed medication or treatment? _____

_____

_____


33) Has the student/resident/individual experienced any significant life events or changes? (ex., family member's or friend's death, traumatic event, recent move, parental divorce, foster care)

_____

_____

_____


Function: Tell the person you are interviewing, "The function of the behavior is the purpose it serves the student/resident/individual. It can be broken down into two purposes–to gain/obtain or to escape/avoid."

34) What purpose does the behavior serve? What do you think he/she is trying to gain or avoid?

_____

_____

_____


Interventions: There are behavioral strategies that the person you are interviewing has most likely tried (example: grounding, behavior charts, stickers, earn money or toy)

35) What have you tried to help improve the behavior? Any strategies? Any interventions?

_____

_____

_____


36) What has been effective? What has worked? _____

_____

_____


37) What has been ineffective? What has not worked? _____

_____

_____

**Preferences:** Personal preferences are especially important in Phase Three: Planning. In the warm-up questions, some of this was introduced. This is a chance for the person being interviewed to reconsider and add more depth to this area (example: computer time, drawing time, five-minute time to just chill out, homework pass, a game with a friend, lunch with the principal, talk time with the teacher, earn points to earn a prize).

38) When you think about rewards or positive reinforcers, what does the student/resident/individual enjoy? _____

_____

_____

39) When you think about rewards or positive reinforcers, what does the student/resident/individual dislike? _____

_____

_____

40) What are some of his/her favorite things? _____

_____

_____

Closing–End on a positive note. Offer the person being interviewed the opportunity to add anything that they feel is relevant.

41) Are there any other items you would like to discuss, or you think would be relevant to the student's behavior or improving his/her behavior? _____

_____

_____

Be sure to thank the interviewee for his/her time. Offer contact information to the interviewee.

# Appendix E

**Functional Behavioral Assessment**
**Phase One: Process**
**Staff/Personnel Interview Questionnaire**

**Student Name:** _____          **Date:**_____

**Adults, Staff Present (Name and Title):**

_____

_____

_____

**Target Behavior(s):** _____

_____

Please use the individual's name in the place of student/resident/individual.

**Warm-Up Questions:** In this first phase of the interview, focus on more neutral topics. The information in the warm-up questions can be revisited in Phase Three: Planning.

1) Please describe your relationship with the student/resident/individual? _____

_____

2) What is a typical day like with him/her? _____

_____

3) Given what you know about the student/resident/individual of him/her, would you please

name some of his/her favorite things to do? (ex., Games, Activities, Talents, Sports, Interests)

_____

_____

4) Name some qualities about him/her. (ex., Friendly, Outgoing, Loyal, Honest, Compassionate)

_____

_____

5) Are there any awards or achievements that he/she has received? (ex., Honor Roll, Sports

Recognition, Chorus Recognition) _____

_____

**Target Behavior Questions:** In this phase of the interview, focus on the target behavior. If there are other behaviors that seem to be more pervasive or challenging in the environment, be sure to investigate these as well.

6) **Characteristics:** Describe the act or actions that the student/resident/individual exhibits that are interfering, disruptive or problematic. Which behaviors seem to be atypical, inappropriate, interfering, uncontrolled, and/or dangerous? If the person being interviewed uses vague descriptions (aggressive, emotion words) redirect and ask them to describe the behavior (hits with fist, runs from classroom, yells verbal threats, such as "I'll kill you!") _____

_____

_____

_____

_____

7) **Pervasiveness:** Tell me more about the student's/resident's/individual's behavior. Prompt questions for clarification: How frequently does the behavior occur? (This can range from multiple times in an hour to monthly.) How intense is the behavior? (This can range from mildly disruptive to causing physical injury to someone.) Finally, what is the duration of the behavior? (This can range from a few seconds to ongoing throughout the entire day.) If there is more than one target behavior, gather this data on each of the behaviors. _____

_____

_____

_____

**Environmental Conditions:** Tell me more about the environmental factors that surround these behavior(s).

8) Where does the behavior occur? What is the setting? (ex., inside the classroom, on the playground, in the office, in the cafeteria, in the hallway, in group therapy, and/or on the jobsite)

_____

_____

_____

9) Is there any place that he/she does not like to be? Is there a place that angers or frightens the student/resident/individual? _____

_____

_____

10) Is there any place that he/she likes to be? Is there a place that the student/resident/individual enjoys or looks forward to attending? _____

_____

_____

11) Who is present when the behavior occurs? (ex., peers, teachers, parents, administrative staff, and/or paraprofessionals) _____

_____

_____

12) Is there anyone he/she likes to be around? Who are his/her friends? _____

_____

_____

13) Does anyone trigger the student's/resident's/individual's behavior? Provoke the behavior?

_____

_____

_____

14) When does the behavior occur? (ex., morning, afternoon, a specific time, or even a specific season) _____

_____

_____

15) Is there a time when the behavior never occurs? (ex., morning, afternoon, a specific time, or even a specific season) _____

_____

16) What is typically happening when this behavior(s) occurs? What are the events or activities taking place? (example: math, reading, transitioning, asked to do a specific task) _____

_____

_____

17) What types of activities or events does the student/resident/individual enjoy? _____

_____

_____

18) What types of activities or events does the student/resident/individual dislike? _____

_____

_____

19) What other triggers can you think of that prompt the behavior of concern?_____

_____

_____

**Respondent Conditions:** The student or resident is considered the respondent.

20) Are there any past or current physiological factors that the student/resident/individual has or is experiencing? (example: mental health issues, illnesses, genetic disorders, chronic conditions and/or other types of impairments or difficulties) _____

_____

_____

21) For a moment, please consider the student/resident/individual. Are there any cultural considerations we should consider? Has he/she always lived in this country? State? Region? Are there any other social rituals, beliefs, language areother differences that he/she experiences?

_____

_____

_____

22) Are there any pharmacological factors that should be considered? Is the student receiving prescribed medication or treatment? _____

_____

_____

23) Has the student/resident/individual experienced any significant life events or changes? (ex., family member's or friend's death, traumatic event, recent move, parental divorce, foster care)

_____

_____

_____

**Function:** Tell the person you are interviewing, "The function of the behavior is the purpose it serves the student/resident/individual. It can be broken down into two purposes–to gain/obtain or to escape/avoid."

24) What purpose does the behavior serve? What do you think he/she is trying to gain or avoid?

_____

_____

_____

**Interventions:** These are behavioral strategies that the person you are interviewing has most likely tried. (ex., behavior charts, stickers, changing color, token economy, discipline referral, suspension)

25) What have you tried to help improve the behavior? Any strategies? Any interventions?

_____

_____

_____

26) What has been effective? What has worked? _____

_____

_____

27) What has been ineffective? What has not worked? _____

_____

_____

**Preferences:** Personal preferences are especially important in Phase Three: Planning. In the warm-up questions, some of this was introduced.This is a chance for the person being interviewed to reconsider and add more depth to this area. (ex., computer time, drawing time, five minute time to just chill out, homework pass, a game with a friend, lunch with the principal, talk time with the teacher, earn points to earn a prize)

28) When you think about rewards or positive reinforcers, what does the student/resident/individual enjoy? _____

_____

_____

29) When you think about rewards or positive reinforcers, what does the student/resident/individual dislike? _____

_____

_____

30) What are some of his/her favorite things? _____

_____

_____

Closing – End on a positive note. Offer the person being interviewed the opportunity to add anything that they feel is relevant.

31) Are there any other items you would like to discuss, or you think would be relevant to the student's behavior or improving his/her behavior? _____

_____

_____

Be sure to thank the interviewee for his/her time. Offer contact information to the interviewee.

# Appendix F

**Functional Behavioral Assessment**
**Phase One: Process**
**Student Questionnaire**

**Student/Resident/Individual Name:** _____**Date:** _____

**Target Behavior(s):** _____

_____

Please use the individual's name in the place of student/resident/individual.

Warm-Up Questions: In this first phase of the interview, focus on more neutral topics. The information in the warm-up questions can be revisited in Phase Three: Planning.

**Relationships:**

1) Tell me about your home. What's your neighborhood like? _____

_____

2) Who lives in your house? _____

_____

3) Do you have any brothers or sisters? If so, how old are they? Do they live in your house?

_____

_____

4) Do you get along with your brothers and sisters? Describe. _____

_____

5) What about everyone else in your home? Do you get along well with them? Or, do you have problems with some or one of them? Describe. _____

_____

6) Who is your favorite family member? What do you like about that person? _____

_____

**Routines:**

7) What is a typical day like for you? What do you do? _____

_____

8) Do you have any chores or household responsibilities? If so, what are they? _____

_____

9) Do you always do your chores when asked? Or, do you get mad or angry about them? If you do, what does that look like? _____

_____

10) Do you have a set bedtime? If yes, what time? _____

11) Do you go to bed when asked or told to? Or, does bedtime become difficult for you? Do you sleep well? _____

_____

12) Are there any other routines or activities that you are required to attend or participate in? Do you like them? Why or why not? If you do not like them, how do you behave? Describe. _____

_____

**Attributes:**

13) What are some of your skills, talents or favorite things to do? (ex., Games, Activities, Talents, Sports, Interests) _____

_____

14) Name some qualities about yourself. (ex., Friendly, Outgoing, Loyal, Honest, Compassionate) _____

_____

15) Have you ever received any awards or special recognition? (ex., Honor Roll, Sports Recognition, Chorus Recognition) _____

_____

**Target Behavior Questions:** In this phase of the interview, focus on the target behavior. If there are other behaviors that seem to be more pervasive or challenging in the environment, be sure to investigate these as well.

**Characteristics:**

16) Tell me about your behavior at home and at school. _____

_____

_____

_____

17) Do you ever get in trouble at home or at school? Describe that to me._____

_____

_____

_____

18) Do adults ever tell you that your behavior is unusual, inappropriate, interfering, uncontrolled, and/or dangerous? (If this is a younger person or cognitively challenged individual, use simpler words. Consider mean, hurtful, mad, a problem, unkind, unfair, wrong, not right) If the person being interviewed uses vague descriptions (aggressive, emotion words) redirect and ask them to describe the behavior (hits with fist, runs from classroom, yells verbal threats, such as "I'll kill you!") _____

_____

_____

_____

_____

19) How do your parents feel about your behavior? How do other family members feel about your behavior? Do they get sad or mad about your behavior? _____

_____

_____

_____

20) How do your teachers feel about your behavior? Do they get sad or mad about your behavior? _____

_____

_____

21) How do your classmates feel about your behavior? Do they get sad or mad about your behavior? _____

_____

_____

22) How do you feel about your behavior? Do you like it? _____

_____

_____

23) Are there times you wish you could change your behavior? When? _____

_____

_____

24) Fill in the blank: When I am angry I _____

25) Fill in the blank: When I am sad I_____

26) Fill in the blank: When I am hurt I _____

27) Fill in the blank: When I am scared I _____

28) Fill in the blank: When I am confused I _____

29) Pervasiveness: If the individual has told you about the target behavior say, "Remember you told me that you sometimes (insert behavior). Can you tell me some more about that. If the individual has not told you about the target behavior yet say, "I know that sometimes you have difficulty. I know that you (insert a simple summary of the target behavior). Let's talk more about that now. Prompt questions for clarification: How often does the behavior occur? (This can range from multiple times in an hour to monthly.) How intense is the behavior? (This can range from mildly disruptive to causing physical injury to someone.) Finally, what is the duration of the behavior? (This can range from a few seconds to ongoing throughout the entire day.) If there is more than one target behavior, gather this data on each of the behaviors. _____

_____

_____

_____

**Environmental Conditions:** Tell me more about the environmental factors that surround these behavior(s).

30) Now, about the behavior we are discussing, where does the behavior occur? What is the setting? (ex., inside the house, in the community, at church, in the living or common area of the home, at a neighbor's house) _____

_____

_____

31) Is there any place you do not like to go? Is there a place that angers or frightens you? _____

_____

_____

32) Is there any place that you like to go? Is there a place that you enjoy or looks forward to attending?_____

_____

_____

33) Who is present when the behavior occurs? (example: parents, stepparents, siblings, step-siblings, grandparents, other family members, neighbors,and/or strangers)_____

_____

_____

34) Is there anyone you like to be around? Who are your friends? _____

_____

_____

35) Does anyone trigger you? Provoke the behavior? _____

_____

_____

36) When does the behavior occur? (ex., morning, afternoon, a specific time, or even a specific season) _____

_____

_____

37) Is there a time when the behavior never occurs? (ex., morning, afternoon, a specific time, or even a specific season) _____

_____

38) What is typically happening when this behavior(s) occurs? What are the events or activities taking place? (ex., chores, bed/bath-time, sports, playing games) _____

_____

_____

39) What types of activities or events do you enjoy? _____

_____

_____

40) What types of activities or events do you dislike? _____

_____

_____

41) What other triggers can you think of that prompt your behavior? _____

_____

_____

**Respondent Conditions:** The student or resident is considered the respondent. If the student cannot answer questions regarding this section, follow up with parents/caregivers/teachers.

42) Do you have an illness or condition that you know about or can talk about? _____

_____

_____

43) Tell me about your heritage. Do you or anyone in your home speak a different language? Describe. Have you lived in this area long? Where else have you lived? _____

_____

_____

44) Do you take any medicine or go for any type of treatment? _____

_____

_____

45) Have you had any recent changes in your family or to any close friends? _____

_____

_____

**Function:** Tell the person you are interviewing, "The function of the behavior is the purpose it serves you. It can be broken down into two purposes – to gain/obtain or to escape/avoid."

46) In talking about your behavior (remind the individual specifically about the target behavior), what purpose does the behavior serve you? Are you trying to gain or avoid something?

_____

_____

_____

**Interventions:** There are behavioral strategies that the person you are interviewing has most likely received. (ex., grounding, behavior charts, stickers, disciplinary forms)

47) Has anyone tried to help you improve your behavior? What have they tried? Any strategies? Any interventions? _____

_____

_____

48) What did you like? What has worked? _____

_____

_____

49) What did you not like? What has not worked? _____

_____

_____

**Preferences:** Personal preferences are especially important in Phase Three: Planning. In the warm-up questions, some of this was introduced. This is a chance for the person being interviewed to reconsider and add more depth to this area (ex., computer time, drawing time, five minute time to just chill out, homework pass, a game with a friend, lunch with the principal, talk time with the teacher, earn points to earn a prize). Consider a personal preference inventory as well.

50) If you had a chance to earn a reward for improved behavior, what would it be? Name several reasonable items, activities, etc._____

_____

_____

51) What types of items, activities, etc. would you NOT want to see? _____

_____

_____

52) What are some of your favorite things? _____

_____

_____

Closing – End on a positive note. Offer the person being interviewed the opportunity to add anything that they feel is relevant.

53) Are there any other items you would like to discuss, or you think would be relevant to the improving your behavior? _____

_____

_____

Be sure to thank the interviewee for his/her time. Offer contact information to the interviewee.

# Appendix G

**Functional Behavioral Assessment**
**Phase One: Process**
**Interview Checklist**

**Contacting Interviewee Checklist:**
__ Purpose of Call
__ Role of Interviewer
__ Role of Interviewee
__ Allowed for Questions
__ Interpreter, Child Assist Personnel or Any Other Individuals Needed at Interview
__ Set an accessible, place, date and time _____

**Prior to Interview: (Preparations for Location/Meeting)**
__ Contacted Responsible Building Personnel (Principal, Teacher or Building Manager)
__ Secured a Meeting Place for Date and Time
__ Informed Any Necessary Parties of Meeting Place, Date and Time
__ Secured Interpreter, Child Assist Personnel or Any Other Individuals Needed

**Information Gathering:**
__ Student Academic Records
__ Disciplinary Records
__ Anecdotal Records
__ Notes
__ Referral Information including Target Behaviors
__ Medical History/Information
__ Other
__ Checklist, Questionnaire, Survey or Other Tools Needed for Interview

**Setting the Atmosphere: (Room)**
__ Comfortable Room Temperature
__ Comfortable Space
__ Appropriate Size for Number of People Present
__ Light Refreshments (Mints, Beverages, etc.)
__ Appropriate Lighting
__ Needed Items (Tissues, Napkins, Pen, Paper, etc.)

**Setting the Atmosphere: (Interviewer Responsibilities)**
__ Introductions
__ Brief Explanation of Credentials
__ Brief Explanation of Role
__ Purpose of Interview
__ Confidentiality
__ Allow for Questions Prior to Beginning

# Appendix H

**Functional Behavioral Assessment**
**Phase One: Process**
**ABC Data Collection Sheet**

**Student Name:** _____          **Date:**_____

**Observation Site:** _____

**Adults, Staff Present (Name and Title):**

_____

_____

_____

**Activity(s) (ex. Independent work, job training, test, group discussion):**

_____

_____

**Target Behavior:** _____

| Time | Antecedent | Behavior | Consequence |
|------|-----------|----------|-------------|
|      |           |          |             |
|      |           |          |             |
|      |           |          |             |
|      |           |          |             |
|      |           |          |             |
|      |           |          |             |
|      |           |          |             |
|      |           |          |             |
|      |           |          |             |
|      |           |          |             |
|      |           |          |             |

**Functional Behavioral Assessment**
**Phase One: Process**
**ABC Data Collection Sheet (Continuation)**

Target Behavior: _____

| Time | Antecedent | Behavior | Consequence |
|------|-----------|----------|-------------|
|      |           |          |             |
|      |           |          |             |
|      |           |          |             |
|      |           |          |             |
|      |           |          |             |
|      |           |          |             |
|      |           |          |             |
|      |           |          |             |
|      |           |          |             |
|      |           |          |             |
|      |           |          |             |
|      |           |          |             |
|      |           |          |             |
|      |           |          |             |
|      |           |          |             |
|      |           |          |             |
|      |           |          |             |

# Appendix I

**Functional Behavioral Assessment**
**Phase Two: Purpose**
**Data Analysis Worksheet**

**Name:** _____     **Date:** _____

**Source: Type/Position/Name** _____

| Records | Parent/Caregiver | Staff | Direct Observation |
|---|---|---|---|
| ___ IEP | ___ Biological | ___ Teacher | Type of Data |
| ___ Disciplinary Report | ___ Foster | ___ Administrator | |
| ___ 504 Plan | ___ Other | ___ Counselor | |
| ___ RTI | Name: | ___ Paraprofessional | |
| ___ Bus Referral | | ___ Other | |
| ___ Medical | Interview/Questionnaire | Name: | |
| ___ Attendance | | Interview/Questionnaire | |
| ___ Other | | | |

**Target Behavior:**

_____
_____
_____
_____

| Characteristics: ___ Atypical ___ Inappropriate ___ Interfering ___ Uncontrolled ___ Dangerous |
|---|

Are there times/circumstances/individuals/situations when the target behavior never occurs?

_____
_____
_____
_____

Are there times/circumstances/individuals/situations when the target behavior always occurs?

_____
_____
_____
_____

**Setting Events:**

| Physiological (Medical, Biological) | Cultural (Heritage, Socioeconomic, Religious) |
|---|---|
| | |
| Pharmacological (Medications, Treatments) | Life Events (Recent traumatic event) |

**Contextual Factors:**

| Who (Individuals Present) | What (Events/Occurrence Factors) |
|---|---|
| | |
| When (Time of day, Season) | Where (Setting) |

**Antecedent:** (what happened before the behavior)

<br>
<br>
<br>
<br>

**Consequences:** (what happened after the behavior)

<br>
<br>
<br>
<br>

**Function:** Is the behavior to access, avoid/escape, communicate or gain/obtain?

| Avoid/Escape | Communicate | Gain/Obtain |
|---|---|---|
| Administrator/School Counselor<br>Attention<br>Activity<br>Academic Task<br>Classroom<br>Discipline<br>Instruction<br>Parental Attention<br>Peer Attention<br>Place/Setting<br>Task<br>Teacher/Paraprofessional Attention<br>Work<br>Other: _____ | Anxiety/Concerns<br>Discomfort<br>Dissatisfaction<br>Physical Pain<br>Response to task, work or request<br>Other: _____ | Administrator/School Counselor<br>Attention<br>Activity<br>Parental Attention<br>Peer Attention<br>Place/Setting<br>Situation<br>Teacher/Paraprofessional Attention<br>Work<br>Other: _____ |
| Social Dynamic (Not Attention) | Stimulation | Tangible |
| Power<br>Control<br>Status<br>Revenge<br>Other: _____ | Repetitive Behavior (flapping,<br>pacing, rocking)<br>Discontented/Bored<br>Impulsive behavior<br>Other: _____ | Activity<br>Game<br>Item<br>Money<br>Token<br>Toy<br>Other: _____ |

**Function of Behavior:**

_____
_____
_____
_____

# Appendix J

**Functional Behavioral Assessment**
**Phase Two: Purpose**
**Data Analysis: Summary Worksheet**

Name: _____ Date: _____

Target Behavior: _____

| Source | Avoid/Escape | Communicate | Gain/Obtain | Social Dynamic (Not Attention) | Stimulation | Tangible |
|--------|--------------|-------------|-------------|-------------------------------|-------------|----------|
| Records | | | | | | |
| Parent | | | | | | |
| Staff #1 Math | | | | | | |
| Staff #1 Reading | | | | | | |
| Staff #1 Science | | | | | | |
| Staff #1 | | | | | | |
| Staff #1 | | | | | | |
| Direct Data | | | | | | |

# Appendix K

**Functional Behavioral Assessment**
**Phase Two: Purpose**
**Data Analysis: Direct Observation Summary Worksheet**

Name: _____     Date: _____

Target Behavior: _____

| Observation Dates | Avoid/Escape | Communicate | Gain/Obtain | Social Dynamic (Not Attention) | Stimulation | Tangible |
|---|---|---|---|---|---|---|
| Observation #1 | | | | | | |
| Observation #2 | | | | | | |
| Observation #3 | | | | | | |
| Observation #4 | | | | | | |
| Observation #5 | | | | | | |
| Observation #6 | | | | | | |
| Observation #7 | | | | | | |
| Observation #8 | | | | | | |
| Observation #9 | | | | | | |
| Observation #10 | | | | | | |

# Appendix L

**Functional Behavioral Assessment**
**Phase Two: Purpose**
**Determining the Function Help Chart**

Student Name: _____ Date: _____

Target Behavior:_____

First, ask yourself: *Is the behavior to avoid/escape, communicate, gain/obtain or access?*
Second, choose from the list. If the function is not on the chart, write in your own.

| Avoid/Escape | Communicate | Gain/Obtain |
|---|---|---|
| Administrator/School Counselor Attention Activity Academic Task Classroom Discipline Instruction Parental Attention Peer Attention Place/Setting Task Teacher/Paraprofessional Attention Work Other: _____ | Anxiety/Concerns Discomfort Dissatisfaction Physical Pain Response to task, work or request Other: _____ | Administrator/School Counselor Attention Activity Parental Attention Peer Attention Place/Setting Situation Teacher/Paraprofessional Attention Work Other: _____ |
| Social Dynamic (Not Attention) | Stimulation | Tangible |
| Power Control Status Revenge Other: _____ | Repetitive Behavior (flapping, pacing, rocking) Discontented/Bored Impulsive behavior Other: _____ | Activity Game Item Money Token Toy Other: _____ |

# Appendix M

**Functional Behavioral Assessment**
Process, Purpose, Planning, Prevention

**Student Name:** _____**DOB:** _____**Date:**_____

Participants Present (Name andTitle)

_____        _____
_____        _____
_____        _____
_____        _____
_____        _____
_____        _____

**Process** (List target behavior(s) along with operationalized definitions.)

Target Behavior One:
_____
_____

Target Behavior Two:
_____
_____

Target Behavior Three:
_____
_____

**Data Collection**

**Indirect Assessment:**

| Record Review Summary: Circleall that Apply |
| --- |
| Medical   Assessment   IEP   Disciplinary Reports   Attendance Record   Other: _____ |

Interview Review Summary: Circle all that Apply

Parent/Caregiver/Guardian    Teacher    Special Education Teacher    Counselor    Student
Other: _____

_____
_____
_____
_____
_____
_____
_____
_____
_____
_____
_____
_____

Assessment Summary: Circle all that Apply

Parent/Caregiver/Guardian    Teacher    Special Education Teacher    Counselor    Student
Other: _____

Name(s) of Assessment:

_____
_____
_____
_____
_____
_____
_____
_____
_____
_____
_____
_____

**Direct Observation**

Observation Summary:

**Purpose**

Data Analysis:
_____
_____
_____
_____
_____
_____
_____
_____
_____
_____

TargetBehavior One: _____

Hypothesis Statement:
_____
_____
_____

Explanatory Summary:
_____
_____
_____
_____
_____
_____
_____

Target Behavior Two: _____

Hypothesis Statement:
_____
_____
_____

Explanatory Summary:
_____
_____
_____
_____
_____
_____

Target Behavior Three: _____

| Hypothesis Statement: |
| --- |
|  |
|  |
|  |
|  |
| Explanatory Summary: |
|  |
|  |
|  |
|  |
|  |
|  |
|  |

## **Planning**

Target Behavior One: _____

| Brief Summary of Recommendations: |
| --- |
|  |
|  |
|  |
|  |

Target Behavior Two: _____

| Brief Summary of Recommendations: |
| --- |
|  |
|  |
|  |
|  |

Target Behavior Three: _____

| Brief Summary of Recommendations: |
| --- |
|  |
|  |
|  |
|  |

**Prevention** (Changes made to the environment's climate, culture and community.)

Target Behavior One: _____

| Prevention Plan: |
| --- |
|  |
|  |
|  |
|  |

Target Behavior Two: _____

| Prevention Plan: |
| --- |
| |

Target Behavior Three: _____

| Prevention Plan: |
| --- |
| |

**Meeting date for Behavior InterventionPlanning:**_____

| Other: (concerns,comments, looking ahead statements) |
| --- |
| |

# Appendix N

**Functional Behavioral Assessment**
**Phase Three: Planning**
**Behavior Intervention Plan**

**Student Name:** _____ DOB: _____ Date: _____

Participants Present (Name and Title)

_____        _____
_____        _____
_____        _____
_____        _____
_____        _____
_____        _____

Target Behavior One: _____
_____
_____

Function of Behavior: _____
_____
_____

Antecedent Modifications (List all that apply): _____
_____
_____
_____

Replacement Behaviors: _____
_____
_____
_____

Reinforcers: _____
_____
_____
_____

Consequences: _____
_____
_____
_____

Target Behavior Two: _____
_____
_____

Function of Behavior: _____
_____
_____

Antecedent Modifications (List all that apply): _____
_____
_____
_____

Replacement Behaviors: _____
_____
_____
_____

Reinforcers: _____
_____
_____
_____

Consequences: _____
_____
_____
_____

Target Behavior Three: _____
_____
_____

Function of Behavior: _____
_____
_____

Antecedent Modifications (List all that apply): _____
_____
_____

Replacement Behaviors: _____
_____
_____

Reinforcers: _____
_____
_____

Consequences: _____
_____
_____
_____

Plan of Action (Method of data collection, personnel involved, progress monitoring parameters, reporting):

_____

_____

_____

_____

_____

_____

_____

_____

_____

_____

_____

_____

Progress Monitoring:

Date: _____ Progress: _____

Date: _____ Progress: _____

Date: _____ Progress: _____

Date: _____ Progress: _____

Additional Information: _____

_____

_____

# Index

**A**
ABA, 164
ABC form, 93, 94
ABC *See* Antecedent-behavior-consequence, 11
Advocate, 29, 45, 56
Analysis worksheet, 101, 102, 106
Antecedent, 11, 17, 18, 42, 63, 103, 105, 127, 136, 138
Antecedent-behavior-consequence, 103
Atmosphere setting, 61, 65
Atypical behavior, 40

**B**
Baseline data, 33, 36, 88, 141, 146, 150, 153
Behavior, 3, 9, 10, 14, 16, 33, 40, 45, 47, 51, 85, 114, 124, 134, 135, 138, 142, 138
  definition of, 125
  disruptive, 47
  spectrum of, 79
  standard of, 60
Behavioral intervention plans (BIPs), 13, 141
Behavioral strategies, 12, 39, 65, 132, 145, 151
Behaviorism, 10, 15, 16
Behavior planning, 4–6, 28, 32, 39
  goal of, 40
  parameters of, 145

**C**
Climate, 5, 140, 163, 165, 166
Community, 3, 5, 27, 29, 30, 40, 113, 126, 130, 140, 163, 164
Confidentiality, 30, 54, 57, 62, 65, 74, 85
Consent, 54, 57

Consequence, 5, 11, 13, 15, 16, 18, 45, 63, 103, 126, 127, 135, 149, 151
  application of, 152
Contextual factors, 4, 64, 90, 92, 103, 114–116, 145, 148
Continuous reinforcement, 149
Correlation, 102
Crisis prevention, 165, 166
Culture, 5, 131, 140, 163–166

**D**
Data analysis, 5, 99, 100, 102, 105, 113, 115, 138
Data collecting, 25, 51, 63, 83
Data collection, 27, 51, 52, 143
  form of, 103
  forms of, 74
  method of, 88, 91, 100
  type of, 110
  types of, 59, 83, 87, 92
De-escalation, 165, 166
Descriptive behavior, 33, 92
Direct methods, 51
Duration, 45, 64, 84, 89, 91, 103, 110, 150

**E**
Environmental conditions, 3, 63, 64, 87

**F**
FERPA, 54
Formal assessment, 71–73, 75
  characteristics of, 81
Frequency, 44, 45, 64, 84, 103, 110, 127, 143
Function, 4, 5, 15, 18, 136, 139
  definition of, 9

© Springer International Publishing Switzerland 2016          227
S. M. Hadaway, A. W. Brue, *Practitioner's Guide to Functional Behavioral Assessment*,
Autism and Child Psychopathology Series, DOI 10.1007/978-3-319-23721-3

development of, 25, 27, 61, 71, 83, 86
history of, 9
Functional analysis screening tool (FAST),
74, 127
Functional behavioral assessment (FBA)
definition of, 13
development of, 9, 14, 33

**G**
Graphing, 105

**H**
Hypothesis, 3, 5, 16, 99, 102, 107, 113–116,
139, 145

**I**
IDEA 2004, 12–14, 42, 147, 164
Indirect methods, 52, 83, 100
Individualized education program (IEP), 13,
31, 54, 147
Influencing factors, 146
Informal assessment, 52, 59, 72–74, 83, 99
Intensity, 44, 45, 64, 84, 127, 164
Interfering behavior, 4, 10, 13, 27, 40, 41, 86,
163, 164, 165
Interval reinforcement, 150, 151
Interviews, 25, 32, 33, 35, 39, 52, 99, 100, 127
gained from, 59

**L**
Latency, 91, 105

**M**
Measureable behavior, 35, 40, 66
Motivation assessment scale (MAS), 74

**O**
Observational data, 83, 99, 103
Operational definition, 61, 125, 165
Operationalize behavior, 35, 46
definition of, 46, 125

**P**
Parental consent, 29, 32, 35
Planning, 5, 6, 19, 25, 114, 140, 145, 150,
163, 165

Prediction, 10, 100, 145
Prevention, 4, 5, 19, 114, 131, 140, 148, 163,
164
Primary sources, 62
Privilege, 57
Process, 3, 5, 6, 9, 18, 25, 56, 61, 62, 114, 145
time-consumings, 89
Purpose, 5, 32, 74, 99, 113, 138

**Q**
Qualitative data
types of, 99
Quantitative data, 99
Questionnaires, 25, 33, 59, 72, 101, 126
Questions about behavioral function (QABF),
75

**R**
Rating scales, 77, 127
Ratio reinforcement, 150
Record review, 25, 53
Release
of information, 55, 56, 57
Replacement behavior, 5, 19, 40, 63, 146, 148,
149–151

**S**
Safety planning, 45
Scatter plot, 87, 90
Secondary sources, 52, 59, 83, 102
Setting events, 17, 42, 63, 116
Surveys, 25, 35, 59, 72

**T**
Target behavior, 5, 7, 30, 34, 39, 42–45, 51,
83, 84, 106, 125, 127, 152
definition of, 125
Team members, 27, 29, 33, 35

9 783319 237206